Whole Foods for You

by Lee Fryer & Dick Simmons

WHOLE FOODS FOR YOU

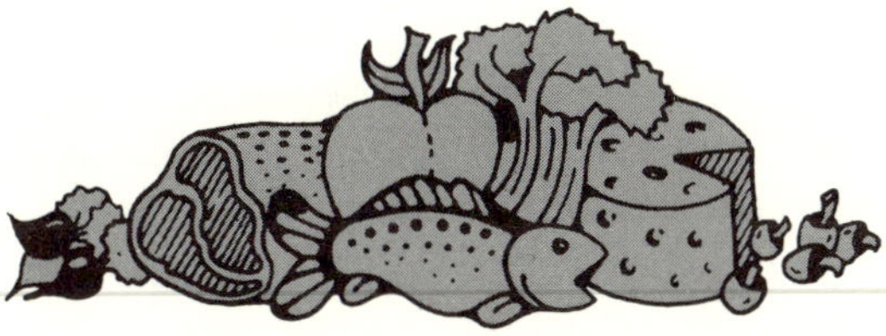

with

Sprouts & Recipes

by Catharyn Elwood

Foreword by Euell Gibbons

Graphics by Christine Becker *and* Ruby Krassner

Mason & Lipscomb PUBLISHERS NEW YORK

ISBN: 0-88405-079-3
Library of Congress Catalog Card Number:
Printed in the United States of America

First Printing

Whole Foods for You

is dedicated to

Marian Fryer.

She provided whole foods

for the authors.

CONTENTS

FOREWORD

Everywhere people demand, "Give us some simple rule which, if followed, will assure us of an adequate, healthful diet." There are many such rules around, the only trouble is they don't work. Have you encountered negative food faddism – the attempt to merely exclude certain categories of food?

"Don't eat packaged food" – as if a food changed its nature if put into a bag to carry it home. Some packages are wasteful, polluting, and deceitful, but let's not refuse to eat eggs because the hen delivers them nicely packaged in a shell.

"Don't eat processed foods" is almost as ridiculous. Certainly some foods are subjected to harmful processes which remove some of the nutrients, but unless we are to return to grazing our food on hands and knees, we must process it. Threshing grain is a process; grinding it is a process. Most of the food in health food stores has been subjected to one or more processes.

"Avoid everything chemical" won't work because nature herself is the greatest of chemists, building extremely complex compounds from simpler compounds and elements. Without this chemistry we would all die of starvation.

Even such a widely accepted cliche as "Eat only natural foods and you will be alright" will not work. I know some natural foods which contain natural poisons that will kill you just as dead as any industrial product ever manufactured.

Of course, what these people are asking is: "How can I be sure of having a healthful diet without learning anything about foods or nutrition?" Sadly, I have had to reply, "You can't."

I'm not impressed when people say, "My grandmother fed her family alright and she never heard of vitamins or minerals." She probably fed her family better than you ever will, even if you do learn all about foods and nutrition, because all she had available were fresh garden-grown vegetables, her own chickens and eggs, milk fresh from the family cow, meat from animals fattened exactly to their own taste and home-butchered and the meat home-cured, fresh-ground grains from her own family's farm, and a vast knowledge of the wild game, fish, wild fruits and wild vegetables which formed an important part of country people's diet at that time. How could she not give her family a good diet?

I don't mean everyone has to become a nutritionist and a dietician, but they will have to learn enough to understand what these specialists are saying. When those perfectly willing to learn asked me where they should begin, I could not, until now, give a very satisfactory answer. I would hesitate to offer to the general reader the dry tomes and tables which I studied for years while learning enough to write my books. Now comes WHOLE FOODS FOR YOU by Lee Fryer and Dick Simmons, the answer we needed.

This is not just another pair of health food freaks; indeed they deplore the polarization into health-food people and non-health-food people. They want to see everyone eating better food and thereby enjoying better health. They recognize that modern agriculture, the food industry and the supermarket system of distribution are necessary to feed our vast population. They want to teach the shopper to get better food through the regular systems of distribution, and by his selection bring pressure to get better food offered to him.

Written in simple, non-technical language are easily followed directions on how to get whole, healthful foods at economical prices. And who said that learning about foods and nutrition had to be a chore? The authors have fun with food and their enjoyment is contagious. You may start reading this book out of a sense of duty, but you will finish it for the pleasure of reading it.

Euell Gibbons

ACKNOWLEDGMENTS

Earth & Sea Products, Inc. of Santa Cruz, California, added depth and beauty to this book by providing resources for research and graphics.

Robert Swann and **International Independence Institute,** Ashby, Massachusetts, helped with the financing arrangements and promotion.

Food & Earth Services, Inc., Wheaton, Maryland, and Roger Wilks assisted with business and office services.

Rural Advancement Fund, Charlotte, North Carolina, assisted with studies of special fertilizers to produce mineral-rich foods, and with studies of seaweed materials as nontoxic pest controls.

Morton Katz of Ecology Mart, Silver Spring, Maryland, and his staff assisted in assessments of food oils and vitamin and mineral supplements.

Thomas Lipscomb, president, Mason & Lipscomb Publishers, provided creative publishing services, with the aim that *Whole Foods for You* might be suitable for distribution in supermarkets as well as in conventional book markets.

Sy Gresser, editor and writer, provided day and night assistance in mobilizing research materials for the book.

Whole Foods for You

This book concerns a widespread American problem: how to select foods for health and good eating, even in the Supermarket Age. High and rising food prices add, of course, to this problem. Food shoppers need useful new guides to better foods and nutrition for their money.

We show in this chapter what has happened to American foods in the past 30 years, so we may commence discussing your problems *in selecting whole foods for good eating.*

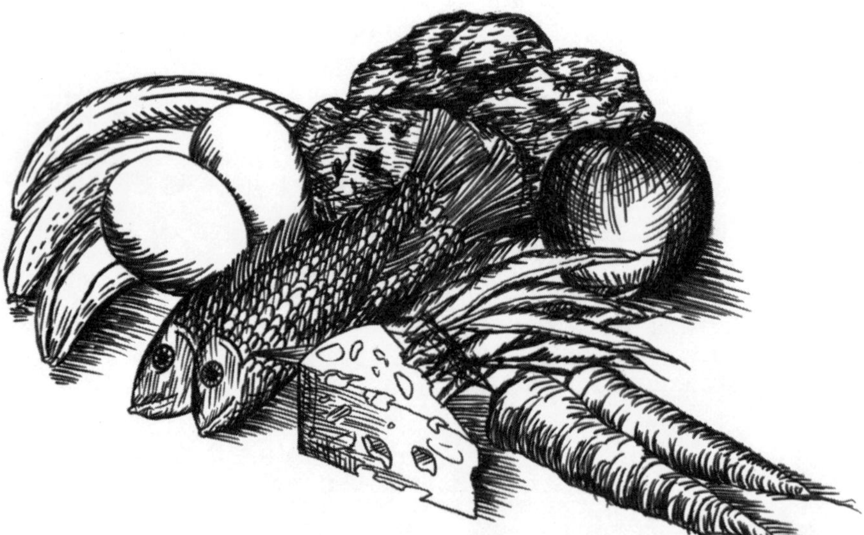

Your Personal Food Guide

When lettuce rises to 40¢ a head, it suddenly becomes important as to whether or not to buy it, and whether it contains food values that are really essential for you.

The books say that lettuce contains iron to prevent iron-deficiency anemia and vitamin A for your general health. As the price of lettuce rises, consumers begin to ask: How much iron and vitamin A does regular head lettuce contain, in these days of high-speed farming? Is "organic" lettuce better, and worth more for the money? Is green-leafed lettuce (romaine and other green kinds) a better buy, from a nutritional standpoint, than regular iceberg head lettuce? And if lettuce at 40¢ a head isn't worth the price, what else can people buy that tastes good and still provides essential vitamins and food minerals?

For many food shoppers, it has become time to know, since they can no longer afford to buy lettuce and other salad vegetables simply as table decorations or as tokens of good family nutrition. In these high-priced times, tokens of good nutrition must also be economical.

In the case of meats, the food shopper's problem is even more complex. Meats, fish, and poultry contain key nutrients that we surely need: protein, iron, other food minerals, vitamins, and good fats. But the price! Two dollars a pound for good red meats, and still going up, with the prospect that economical meats, fish, and poultry are gone forever. What can people do when these vital foods – the meal-builders in most American homes – move out of reach due to high prices? What about the meat helpers, meat-flavored rice, soya-meats, and other substitutes on the supermarket shelves? Are they worth the money?

What will happen to millions of children, young people, and snack eaters – who live on hamburgers, hot dogs, and meat sandwiches – as the food industry takes the meat out of hamburgers and other kinds of sandwiches and puts in tasty substitutes? Is textured vegetable protein (TVP) an acceptable substitute to mix with meats or to eat instead of meat?

And the fruits and juices, what a jungle! Oranges and grapefruits contain precious vitamin C, plus cargoes of vital food minerals. But good oranges are often 8¢ apiece and pasteurized juice is 60¢ a quart. As alternatives, we have canned and frozen juices, with bona fide values. Beyond these, however, are canned punch, frozen punch, "High C," and many other imitation fruit drinks and breakfast beverages, usually laced with sugar and a bit of factory-made vitamins. Are these fruit substitutes worth the money, or even worth carrying home? Should thoughtful mothers corrupt their children's diets with these imitation foods?

These are vital questions of our food times.

We hope this book will help you to cope with some of these present-day food questions and problems. We will try to look at food shopping through the eyes of America's 60 million homekeepers who are trying to use good sense in selecting supermarket foods. We hope that it will serve as an intelligent guide for buying nutritional foods in our Supermarket Age, when many grocery products have been devitalized. Most of all, this is a personal guide to help you in selecting your own foods for good health and good eating.

How times change

Only 30 years ago, the suggestions in this book would have been unnecessary. First, there were no supermarkets as we know them today, although very large grocery stores had come into being. The nation's foods were being sold mainly in about

391,000 local food markets, scattered everywhere people lived. Typical grocery stores had from 1,000 to 3,000 square feet of space (about the same as a modern, four-bedroom house), and they were, in truth, often run by "mama and papa." The food items in these stores were fairly unmolested and uncomplicated, such as people had been buying and eating for many years. A degree in home economics was not needed in order to tell the difference between various kinds of hamburger or breakfast foods.

Also only 30 years ago, 6 million independent, family-type farmers were scattered throughout America, producing food crops and products in a medium-speed farming system. It was modified "organic" farming, since only small amounts of fertilizers and farm chemicals were being used, compared with today's chemical additives.

Many market gardeners were producing fruits and vegetables near the cities in those days, and in season, fresh and tasty tomatoes, lettuce, melons, plums, apples, berries, and other items could be purchased. The nearby dairymen and poultrymen were supplying fresh milk, butter, chickens, and eggs daily into the local markets.

The drastic changes in this earlier U.S. food system commenced in 1945–1950, just after World War II. We seem to have transferred many of the methods and systems of the big war into our domestic economy. Although large food chains such as A&P, Acme, and Kroger were in full operation prior to 1900, the gigantic food supermarkets as we know them today began to develop in the late '30's, and after World War II. Kroger had over 2,000 stores by 1950. By 1973, annual sales of Safeway, Kroger, Food Fair, Acme, and A&P ranged from 1 to 6 billion dollars. Today, supermarkets account for the sale of more than 85% of all foods.

The supermarkets acted as magnets to attract truckloads, carloads, and then trainloads of uniform, low-priced crops and foods from the nation's farms and food factories into huge superstores, in mass displays such as we see today. Expansion has been so great that experts in the supermarket industry believe there is no supermarket trade left to exploit. The coming of these markets was a revolutionary event, which drastically changed farming, food processing, and our whole national food supply system. This revolutionary event is still happening today.

The following information indicates some of the drastic changes:

(Four million independent farmers have been rubbed out since 1945 (two-thirds of them), reducing costs to be sure, but also drastically changing the character and quality of the farm-produced foods.

(Most of the local market gardeners, dairymen, and poultrymen are no longer in business; foods have to be shipped farther and processed more heavily than they were at any time in our history.

(About 229,000 independent local grocery stores (about 60%) have been closed since 1950, as the supermarket system has grown. Meantime, thousands of dissatisfied food shoppers have flocked to health food stores, trying to find good foods for flavor as well as for health.

(Most of our country's vegetable production has been moved into only four states: California, Arizona, Texas, and Florida. These states now produce over 70% of all U.S. vegetables, using high-speed mass farming methods.

(The use of simplified commercial fertilizers (NPK types) has risen by 1,800%. Many foods have consequently become demineralized and devitalized, due to unbalanced fertilization in their production.

(The use of farm chemicals and toxic pesticides has risen by over 600%. Many foods have consequently become bad inputs to our bodies. For example, beef and chicken livers can no longer be suggested as good sources of iron to cope with iron deficiencies in our diets. Too often, the livers contain dangerous residues of pesticides and growth stimulants used in livestock and poultry farming. Other foods must now be selected and eaten to assure sufficient mineral and vitamin intake for our needs.

In terms of a food revolution, American food shoppers, since 1950, have been forced to accept less vital nourishment for their money. The demineralization and devitalization of the food crops, in themselves, are giving consumers less food for their money and will compel certain changes in our food shopping choices if we are to be fed adequately.

New guides are needed. It is not enough simply to point out that livers are often polluted and that children's breakfast foods are often overprocessed, oversugared and, debased – as well as very high priced. It is more important to know what else to buy in a personal and family program of sound nutrition and good eating, still within budget limits.

Actually, when you walk through the food market doors, you enter a new world of foods. This is the food revolution in action. You may choose, for example, from the following different classes of foods:

¶ **Debased foods** such as "filled" and "extended" wieners, sausages, cheese, lunch meats, patties and soyaburgers, and sugar-filled breakfast cereals.

¶ **Demineralized foods,** such as agribusiness lettuce, carrots, tomatoes and corn, grown without sufficient mineral fertilization.

¶ **Imitation foods,** such as High C breakfast drinks, made from sugar, water, fruit concentrate, ascorbic acid, and coloring matter.

¶ **Enriched foods,** such as bread and breakfast cereals, "enriched" with iron and vitamins.

¶ **Fortified foods** such as bread "fortified" with lysine (an amino acid very important in human chemistry).

¶ **Diet foods** such as low-sugar canned goods, cola drinks, and sodas.

¶ **Textured foods,** such as textured vegetable proteins (TVP), in which soybeans are spun like rayon and offered as meat (protein) substitutes.

¶ **Natural foods** such as vitamin C pills made from rose hips or acerola (the Caribbean cherry).

- **Synthetic foods,** such as vitamin C in the form of manufactured ascorbic acid.

- **Organic foods,** such as fruits and vegetables, grown with manures, composts, and earth minerals rather than with commercial fertilizers.

- And of course, **polluted foods,** such as chickens raised with arsenic, antibiotics, and stilbestrol . . . or ham and lunch meats embalmed with sodium nitrate.

May we agree, in the face of this situation, that it is time for new food shopping guides, so you can pick your way through this food jungle and select particular groceries and food supplements you wish and need in your personal program of good health and good eating?

Whole foods in earlier human history were the whole plants, seeds, and fruits we ate, minus the inedible husks, skins, cores, and other tough tissues that we discarded. Or, the **whole** animals, minus their hair, hooves, claws, bones, and other inedible parts. Or, **whole** birds, eggs, fish, and lizards, minus their tough and scaly parts. We built the human saga on a diversified **whole food** diet, in which we have eaten nearly everything that grows, flies, runs, creeps, crawls, or falls from the sky. The world has been our cafeteria.

The hazard of supermarkets is that they threaten to defeat man's ability to glean **whole foods** and put them together into adequate diets. How do you balance out pizzas, sugar pops, and corn kurls and fit them into a mosaic of good foods? How do you build a budget-oriented family diet out of TV dinners, pot pies, hamburger helpers, diet sodas, instant potatoes, fruit loops, and white bread? Can anybody do it?

Our challenge is to run this assortment of present-day supermarket foods through an imaginery sieve and come out with many sensible items that you can choose from and combine in building your own whole food diet.

Whole Foods for You will attempt to provide such useful suggestions and guides. It may help you to survive, feel good and be reasonably happy, even in a Supermarket World.

FOODGRAM No. 1

Combine your foods for low-cost protein

Is Meat Too High-Priced to Eat Every Day?

Then combine seeds and cereals for high-quality protein at low cost in many meals.

Rice and beans are a good example. Separately, they have only medium protein values, but **together**, they make a high-value food. This is a sample comparison with meat:*

		Protein value is equal to:
A.	Eaten separately	
1 ½	cups of cooked brown rice	**7 oz. steak**
4	cups cooked beans (or peas)	**6¼ oz. steak**
	Total	**13¼ oz. steak**
B.	When eaten together	
1 ½	cups rice **plus**	**19 oz. steak**
4	cups beans	
	Increase in protein value	**43%!**

Reason for the increase: The amino acids in the different cereals and grains combine to make high-quality proteins, often equal to meat. Adding a bit of fish or poultry to these lower-cost foods also promotes their total food values. Millions of people over the world have been using such wisdom for centuries. Note their basic country recipes: Beans and corn (Mexico and Latin America), rice and a bit of fish (Japan and Polynesia), and rice and soybeans (China).

Other examples of low-cost protein food combinations:

	Increase in protein value when eaten together
Soybeans and rice	24%
Rice and milk	29%
Whole wheat (bread) and cheese	25%
Corn and beans (in various cooked forms)	50%
Peanuts and sunflower seeds	19%

Later in **Whole Foods for You**, we will give recipes for some of these money-saving food combinations.

* Based on information given in Frances Moore Lappe. *Diet for a Small Planet.* New York: Ballantine Books. 1971.

The importance of whole foods to mankind is that people have been eating such foods for millions of years. We cannot predict what will occur in peoples' systems, particularly Americans', if our diets are subdivided from healthy nutrients and supplied with substitutes which are without nourishment, in some cases harmful, and above all, expensive.

We get a perspective in this chapter on where we stand in relation to our food supplies – today with supermarkets, compared with 40 years ago . . . and 4,000 years ago . . . and even 4 million years ago. Doing this is useful if we are to select foods for good nutrition at low costs.

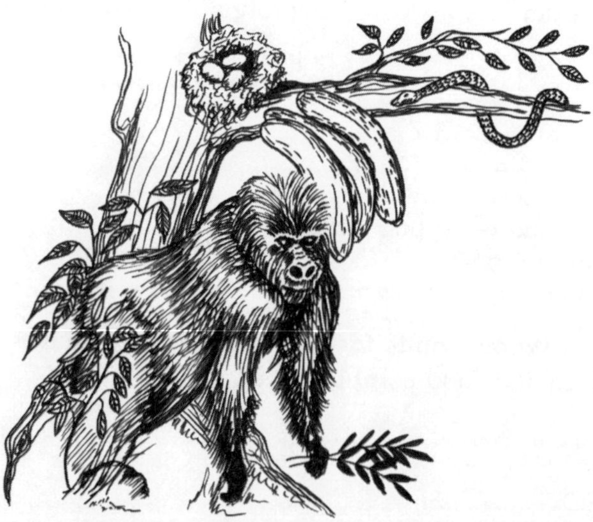

1

The Human Food Calendar

During the period in human evolution when our ancestors began living primarily upon the land, the human diet changed radically. Up in the trees, they probably ate tender shoots, fruits, birds' eggs, nestlings, bugs, and occasional squirrels and lizards. On the ground, they learned to eat roots, vegetables, snakes, turtles, sweet flowers, mice, insects, birds, small animals, fish, seeds, grains, honey, and fruits and berries. Eventually, man also learned to kill and eat larger animals.

There is evidence that we have built into our personal food systems many of the minerals and food factors that existed along our evolutionary pathways. Where there was salt, a need for salt evolved, and it was used. Where there was iron, we seized it and formed our enzymes around the bits of iron – or zinc, copper, cobalt, and three dozen other minerals active in our environment. Where sugar was present in the tissues of our early foods, we took it and built a metabolic system in our bodies to convert the sugar into energy.

We consumed amino acids in the plants and creatures we ate and used these precious protein food blocks, ready-made, in synthesizing our own personal proteins for muscles and growth.

In the case of vitamins, so essential to mental and physical health, we learned to make many of these in our own bodies from various minerals and protein units in our foods, with the help of our enzymes. However, where our natural foods such as fruits and vegetation were filled with such a vitamin as vitamin C, no need existed to make this vitamin within our bodies; therefore, we never learned to do it. People are still wholly dependent upon daily foods for their vitamin C supplies.

According to Dr. Linus Pauling, gorillas ordinarily get about 4,000 milligrams of vitamin C a day in their foods. A man-sized gorilla, half as big as a fully grown one, might consume about 2,000 milligrams of vitamin C each day. These data cast doubt on the view of the Food and Drug Administration that people need only about 60 milligrams of vitamin C a day – less than 1/30 as much as a person may have consumed during an earlier period of human history.

Humans developed a gut and gastronomic system over 20 feet long during the past 4 million years because dozens of different kinds of foods were eaten. None of these foods resembled hot dogs, sodas, pizzas, potato chips, and TV dinners. An intestinal tract 5 feet long is surely sufficient to handle those kinds of foods.

Only God knows what will happen to people when the terminal 15 feet of their digestive systems no longer need to be used. It is too early in man's unique history to make an accurate guess but the prospects appear gloomy. As a useful panorama of what is happening to people regarding their foods, let us look at a "Human Food Calendar." It will serve to give us more patience with doctors, nutritionists, grocers, food companies, and public officials who are also lost and wandering about in America's big food swamp.

To dramatize this picture of people and their foods coming down the corridors of history, imagine 4,000 trucks moving along – with each truck carrying the foods people ate for 1,000 years. Then, 3,900 trucks would drive by before the first one with any cooked foods on it; 3,995 before the first one with any bread on it; and 3,999 before one had any nonorganic foods on it. The very last truck would have a dab of supermarket groceries in its cargo. Just a dab, that's all.

People were produced with whole foods. Our diets during thousands of years were fairly adequate and balanced because we ate the assortments of elements that prevail in nature – our historical environment.

It was impossible for us to get a bite of iron, during these long years, without also getting biologically balanced intakes of manganese, zinc, copper, cobalt, iodine, silver,

Human food calendar

Legend: 1 day equals 11,000 years
1 hour equals 460 years
1 minute equals 8 years

Approximate date	What happened	Time, if human history were only one year long
4 million years ago	Our descent from trees, eating all kinds of foods.	365 days (1 year) ago
500,000 years ago	Upright, camp life with use of fire.	45 days ago
100,000 years ago	Roasting and baking some of the foods in campfires; early acts of cooking.	9 days ago
11,000 years ago	Simple farming as an improved way of getting foods.	1 day ago (yesterday)
7,000 years ago	Boiling of vegetables and meats in pots.	15 hours ago
4,500 years ago	Beer invented. Grinding grain regularly and making bread.	10 hours ago
150 years ago	Food canning in tin cans; the dawn of modern food processing.	Only 20 minutes ago
50 years ago	Modern farming, with extensive use of fertilizers and pesticides.	Only 6 minutes ago
25 years ago	Agribusiness farming, heavy food processing, supermarketing of foods; and large scale eating of hot dogs, hamburgers, french fries, sodas, potato chips, TV dinners, instant meals, and snack foods.	Only 3 minutes ago

vanadium, and the entire range of other earth minerals. It was equally impossible for us to receive vitamin E without getting its subtle nutrient companions, such as octacosanols and phosphatides, which also occur in raw vegetable oils.

We are not interested in the mysticism or beauty of these food concepts, but rather in the guides they offer for selecting supermarket groceries that will nourish us adequately, at reasonable costs, today.

No one fully knows what may happen if people stray too far from age-old clusters of nutrients in staple groceries. The recent shifts to debased, demineralized, and polluted foods have not been proven harmful to people by disciplined research; however, it has not been demonstrated that they are acceptable in a society of healthy, productive people. We are not a healthy society in the United States, being increasingly afflicted by degenerative diseases of the heart, lung, gland, brain, stomach, blood, and kidney. The quality of the groceries may be a part of this problem.

No sustained research has been conducted to find out how much of the superprocessed foods can be accepted in our diets before we lose normal health and vitality. Calendarwise, there has not been sufficient time to make reliable observations. We have been eating the superfoods for only 25 years – which is only a heartbeat in the long career of man on Earth.

The relative ignorance about today's foods will not embarrass us as we enter the supermarket doors in our quest for whole foods and good groceries. We do know how these foods were grown and processed and where they came from. On this basis, we can select sound foods and construct a healthy diet: a carrot, a fish, brown rice, good crackers, dried milk, a sweet potato, sunflower seeds, a stewing hen, vitamin C pills, sprigs of parsley, black beans, granola, eggs, wheat germ oil, a can of spinach, whole grain bread, cantaloupes, kelp pills, romaine lettuce, yeast, onions, grain sprouts, cheese, a tomato, wine, a piece of steak – and many more. These are building blocks for use in making good meals, snacks, and personal food programs.

It is possible to continue our long pathway from the Cave Age through the supermarkets and into America's future – as healthy productive people.

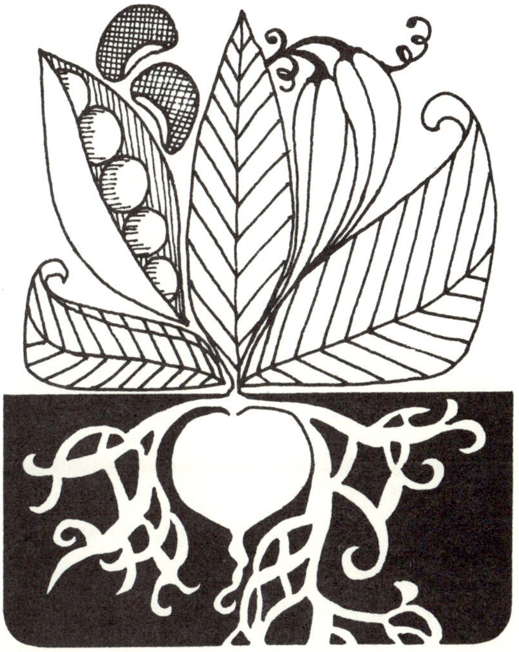

A whole food is a useful building block in a nutritious, economical diet. For its kind, it offers full nutritional values. For example, if it is milk, the cows were properly fed; if it is a chicken, the bird had balanced feeds; if it is corn, the field was fertilized with earth minerals; and if it is lettuce, the green leaves have good levels of iron and vitamin A in the tissues.

Manufacturing and processing did not debase and destroy the food values. For example, the miller kept the bran and germs of wheat in the flour, and the baker made it into whole grain bread. The food oils are lightly processed, so they retain essential raw oil nutrients such as vitamin E and lecithin.

Whole foods are safe to eat. Eventually, they will be systematically sampled and tested in laboratories to see that they do not contain additives, growth stimulants, and toxic residues that are harmful to people. Neither foods nor people can be whole if they are regularly filled with dross materials.

Above all, whole foods must be cheap enough in grocery markets so all people can afford to buy them. America must never become a nation of nutritional haves and have-nots. Democracy in foods is as necessary as the right to vote.

There is no "average" person where foods and nutrition are concerned. We differ from one another in our inherited needs for nutrients and in our tastes and food preferences. In addition, we learn to love and eat personal foods, even when we know they are poor nutrition for our bodies. Sound guides for food selection and personal nutrition should take into account these deep-seated physical and psychological factors that are always at work when people order their meals, choose their snacks, and select their groceries.

We review in this chapter the forces at work in causing us to select foods. A major force, of course, is how much work we are doing, energy we are spending, and foods we need – how hungry we are. Again, major changes have occurred in the past 50 years, and we are eating smaller meals. This, in itself, cuts down our intake of vitamins and minerals – the "protective" foods. This has to be taken into account in present efforts to get properly fed.

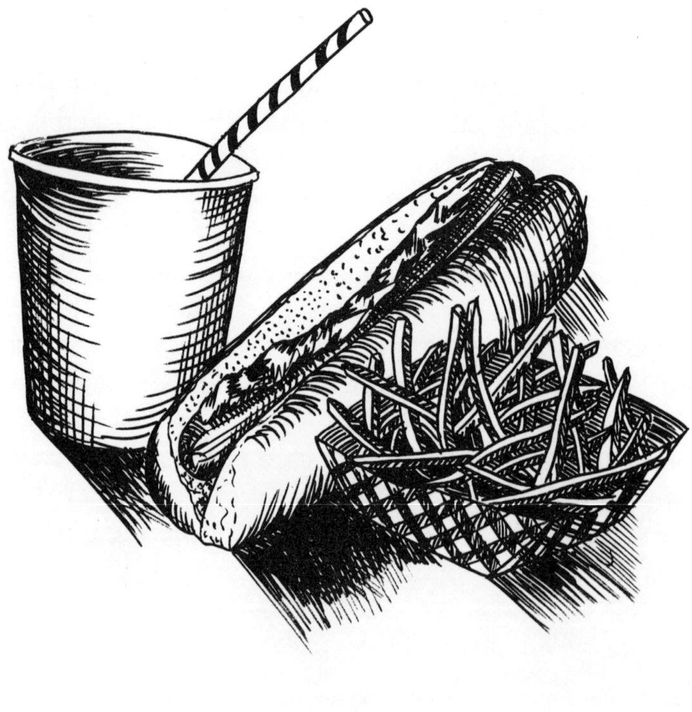

Your Particular Tastes in Foods

If Adam had a brother in the Garden of Eden, it is probable that the brother would not like apples and perhaps would have kept out of trouble. That is the way with people. They are different from one another and have individual tastes in foods. The differences often are basic and physical rather than being simply a matter of training and psychology.

Some people bounce out of bed ready for thoughts and action – and a big breakfast – every day. Others awake by degrees, thinking and moving as little as possible until 10:00 A.M., and more than a cup of coffee and a scrap of toast seems nauseating. Each lives in a specialized food world, and the distinctions are personal, physical and chemical. Ms. A. (the gangbuster type) has a high rate of conversion of her foods into energy – a high rate of metabolism. Ms. B. (the slow-starter type) has a lower metabolic rate and a consequent aversion to foods in the morning hours.

Some people can easily swallow golf balls, while others choke on grapefruit seeds. The difference between their throats is physical, but it may also account for psychological preferences for certain kinds of foods. Also, the narrow-throated person may develop an aversion to taking doctors' prescriptions and food supplement pills.

Dr. Roger Williams has shown that many differences in food tastes and preferences are hereditary – determined in the same fashion as our height, weight, and color of eyes and hair. Also, we have inherited differences in the abilities of our body cells and tissues to receive and use various food elements. Some folks, for example, have difficulty receiving vitamin B_6 and niacin into their brain cells. They consequently need larger amounts of these specific nutrients and may have mental-emotional disorders if the special foods are not provided.

The use of foods and nutrition in the prevention and treatment of diseases is rising as the medical profession learns more about this underresearched field. Leadership and research guidance are being provided by a number of eminent people, including:

Dr. Allan Cott, New York physician-psychiatrist, in use of fasting and special nutrients for treatment of mental-emotional diseases, asthma, and learning disabilities in children.

Dr. Linus Pauling, at Stanford University, in studies of dietary and biochemical needs of people for overcoming various types of illness and sustaining health. He is a research leader in the orthomolecular approach in treating schizophrenia and related mental-emotional disorders.

Dr. Roger Williams, at the University of Texas (Nutrition Against Disease, Bantam Books, 1973, and other books).

Drs. Emanuel Cheraskin and W. H. Ringsdorf, at the University of Alabama (New Hope for Incurable Diseases, Exposition Press, 1971, and other books).

Dr. Carl Pfeiffer, at the New Jersey Neuropsychiatric Institute, in studies of trace mineral nutrition of people in health and disease.

The focus of this pioneer research work is in special needs of many people for particular nutrients, such as vitamins and food minerals, where the underlying cause may be an inherited physical condition. The investigations also shed light on the values of many convenience and snack foods that are finding their way into daily American diets.

Your particular tastes in food

We learn food tastes and preferences, too

In addition to our inherited food needs and tastes, we also learn to love our own personal foods. Good, bad, or horrible, we learn to love them.

Coffee, deep-fried chicken, white bread, ice cream, chocolate puddings, martinis, pork skins, cokes, pancakes and syrup, french fries, candy bars, submarine sandwiches, frosted flakes, donuts, hamburgers, TV beer, pot pies, hot dogs, Danish pastry, potato salad, cheese cake, chitlins, pizzas – you name it, someone loves it; and it is a part of their main eating pattern.

If no one interferes, and if we can afford it, we tend to eat these personal foods. Their selection is often illogical and unwise from the nutrition standpoint, and we know it.

In light of this psychological situation – people's love of their favorite foods – it is often unwise and nonproductive to tell people what they should eat. As a rule, they already know what they should eat, but they cannot find deep-down incentives for choosing the better foods.

Our society and its food industry are responsible, in a large degree, for the poor education and conditioning of people in the selection of their daily foods. The elementary schools fail to educate and orient children sufficiently in nourishment and care of themselves, and in sound food selection. Then, the food industry trains children and older people intensively to select and eat poor foods, via TV and other media advertising. A flagrant example has been the pollution of children's minds and diets with TV commercials that feature sugar-coated breakfast foods and sugar-filled sodas, colas, and other beverages.

Studies by Robert B. Choate (Council on Children, Media and Merchandising) show that TV-viewing children see over 5,000 commercials each year for edible products alone. The ads are often dishonest and misleading in describing the food products, such as breakfast foods; they seldom provide sound nutrition education to the children; often they offer high-cost low-nutrition foods on the basis of leverage appeals, such as games within the package. During one week (ending April 11, 1971), the Broadcast Advertisers' Reports showed that over 50% of the commercials on children's programs were for foods and beverages. As we know, these are usually sugared foods and beverages, and an accumulative effect is generated to teach children that sweet things are good.

This maleducation of children is responsible, in part, for a steady rise in the per capita consumption of sugar in the U.S. from about 96 pounds a year in 1956 to over 115 pounds in 1973. Nearly one-fourth of this increase is in the form of sodas, colas, and other soft drinks. The bad curve is still rising. The average American is eating more than a teaspoon of sugar every 40 minutes, 24 hours a day, 365 days a year.

Many Americans know that a high consumption of sugar, besides causing tooth decay, reduces efficiency in using vitamins and increases susceptibility to diseases. Also, the concentrated starch and sugar foods tend to displace the vitamin, mineral, and protein nutrients in their diets. This substitution inevitably undermines health and lowers resistance to many diseases.

Thousands of young people are reacting to these poor trends as they see the effects of inferior diets on their elders. Many young people want to know about sound, reasonably priced foods and good personal nutrition. They comprise a large portion of the health trade and are joined by at least 5 million diet- and budget-conscious grown-up food shoppers who wish to buy nutritious groceries at fair prices. These sophisticated food customers, young and old, are the leaders in rebuilding personal and national health in the United States.

They are learning to select and like good foods, and to enjoy eating them every day.

The food quantity factor

During 1900 – 1920, Americans often walked when they went places. Otherwise, they rode on horses, in buggies, carriages, and wagons, or on bicycles – occasionally in automobiles, boats, trains, and streetcars. They walked upstairs more often than riding elevators. Adequate exercise was standard and so were big meals. Three thousand calories a day was not unusual, even for slim people.

Workers carried and lifted things – bags, sacks, boxes, steel bars, wood, ice, and coal. Truck drivers loaded and unloaded their cargoes by hand. Stevedores handled 200-pound export bags, and railroad workers loaded 40-ton rail cars by hand. Women cooked large meals and kept house the hard way, without electrical appliances.

Your particular tastes in food

The Western loggers worked 10 hours a day on rough mountain terrain, and their usual foods and diets will serve to illustrate our point that people ate lots of whole foods 50 years ago; the quantity of it, in itself, often assured generous provisions of vitamins and minerals – the key protective foods.

Here is a typical logger's daily fare, 50 years ago:

Breakfast: Stewed prunes, oatmeal, ¼ lb. bacon, 6 eggs, pancakes and syrup, fried potatoes, toast, ham, butter, pie, and coffee with lots of cream and sugar.

Lunch: Four to 6 sandwiches of corned beef, ham and roast meat, beans, jelly, apples, cookies, coffee, and cream and sugar.

Dinner: Steaks, roast, stew, mashed potatoes, gravy, baked beans, onions, carrots, cabbage, string beans, rolls, butter, canned fruit, pie, cake, coffee, and cream and sugar.

This kind of a diet had about 7,000 calories per day. It provided adequate supplies of the protective foods: vitamins, minerals, proteins and good fats. The potatoes alone furnished all of the ascorbic acid (vitamin C) that most people need. The cream, milk, butter, eggs, and carrots took care of vitamins A and D, plus helping with E, B, C, and the food minerals. The meats supplied superprotein nutrition, plus vitamin B, iron, and other bonuses.

It was difficult to be underfed or malfed on such a gross diet. The sheer quantity and variety protected these gargantuan eaters. On the same principle of large meals and diversified foods, millions of other active Americans were fairly well fed 50 years ago.

Now consider a typical 1973 stenographer, GS – 11 administrative assistant, or business executive. These people sleep in cozy places without heat loss. They are transported, elevated, warmed, and cooled throughout their waking hours. The following is a typical daily diet for such people:

Breakfast: 1 glass orange juice or artificial fruit beverage, 2 slices buttered white bread toast, 2 cups coffee with milk and sugar.

Morning Break: 1 soft drink or coffee and 1 donut.

Lunch: 1 white bread or submarine sandwich, 1 piece of pie or pudding, and 1 coffee, beer, or soft drink.

Afternoon Break: 1 soft drink or coffee and potato chips.

Dinner: 1 cocktail, spaghetti and meat balls or a hamburger steak, french fries, 1 vegetable, 1 roll and margarine, dessert, and coffee, tea, or milk.

At Bedtime: A glass of milk, if it was missed at dinner.

The credit card executives will, of course, eat more when they are traveling or entertaining visitors, and the secretaries will eat higher on the hog when they are taken to lunch or dinner by their bosses. These excursions in better eating may serve mainly, however, to fatten the executives and the secretaries rather than improving their diets.

This assortment of foods looks like a good diet, and it is, in fact, a fairly good diet when compared with the daily fare of millions of Americans who do not regularly get fruit juices and high-quality meats. Nevertheless, it is a marginal diet from the standpoint of sound nutrition. There is an analysis on the facing page.

It should be noted that many of these scores are in doubt. Eminent U.S. and foreign nutritionists are in disagreement and controversy as to the amounts of vitamins and minerals that people actually need. Also, leading food advisers disagree concerning the availability of vitamins and minerals: (a) when they are added synthetically to refined foods, such as in enriched white bread, and (b) when they are contained in heavily processed foods, such as vitamin E in heat-treated cooking oils.

Your particular tastes in food

Total intake of foods and beverages 3½ pounds

Total calories		**2,500**
Calories from white flour and sugar	1,250	
Per cent from white flour and sugar	50%	
Total fats		**84 grams**
Hydrogenated vegetable fats	40 grams	
Polyunsaturated vegetable fats	12 grams	
Total vegetable fats	52 grams	
Saturated animal fats	32 grams	
Total fats	84 grams	
Total protein (adequate)		**88 grams**

	Amount	Comments
Calcium (50% is from the milk)	.6 gr.	low
Phosphorus	1 .2 gr.	adequate
Iron (60% is from enriched bread	18 mgrs.	probably low
Other minerals	?	probably low
Vitamin A	4,000 I.U.	low
Vitamin C (40% is from orange juice)	130 mgrs.	low
Thiamin – B_1 (60% is from enriched bread)	1 .7 mgrs.	adequate
Riboflavin – B_2 (50% is from enriched bread)	1 .5 mgrs.	dubious
Niacin	14 .3 mgrs.	dubious
Pyridoxine – B_6	1 .4 mgrs.	dubious
Other vitamins	?	dubious

Dr. Linus Pauling, eminent scientist and nutritionist at Stanford University, commented recently on the disagreements among food scientists as to our needs for vitamin C, and some of his thoughts are given on pages 26 and 27.

Dr. Pauling is making a point that is vital in Whole Foods for You: Marginal nutrition is not enough! Just staying alive and avoiding scurvy, night blindness, rickets, pellagra, and kwashiorkor are not enough! Typical Americans are now seeking guides to a style of living and eating in which their foods will offer greater protection against illness, because this has become financially necessary. Being sick in the U.S. costs too much. Having cancer, heart disease, anemia, and stomach ulcers are personal tragedies; also, they cost too much. The majority of Americans are at the point where they cannot afford the medical, hospital, psychiatric, and dental expenses of everyday living, to say nothing of paying the costs of dread diseases – or for the medical costs of growing old. Even growing old costs too much!

Our groceries and food system, including the quality of farming and the methods of food processing, are a major part of the national health problem. A fresh approach is needed in reexamining the capabilities of sound foods and good nutrition in preventing illnesses – all kinds of illnesses – and keeping people well.

In the chapters that follow, we will assess a number of the major kinds of foods: citrus juices, cooking oils, bread, fruits and vegetables, milk products, meats, meat substitutes, and food supplements. We are keenly aware, in these discussions, of the views of the Food and Drug Administration and the United States Department of Agriculture. We are aware, for example, of their views:

¶ that the nutritive values of food crops are not affected by how those crops are fertilized and grown;

¶ that U.S. foods and diets, generally speaking, are adequate to sustain health;

¶ that dietary supplements of vitamins and minerals are not, generally speaking, needed by Americans to prevent illness and sustain health;

that a heavy processing of foods does not, as a rule, reduce their nutrient values.

Your particular tastes in food

We are aware of the U.S. recommended daily allowances of vitamins and minerals and other key nutrients, published by the Food and Drug Administration, and of its recent actions in limiting the packaging and labeling of dietary foods.

We respect these public food agencies but disagree with some of their views and nutritional guides. They, too, are in transition from an America of 50 years ago when we ate organic foods and walked to our destinations.

A new era of consumerism is emerging in America where people will demand simpler things, less packaging, less overhead costs, less overkill, more honesty in advertising, and more real value for the money. We identify with this new era of consumerism.

You are an extraordinary human being among 4 billion other people on Earth. Food scientists and nutritionists have failed to keep you healthy in their frantic haste to cure your diseases. While engrossed in studying vitamins A, B, C, D, E, and K, individually – and iron, manganese, copper, zinc, iodine, cobalt, and selenium, individually – and all of the amino acids, fats, and sugars, individually – they have failed to study the many nutrients in clusters, families, and galaxies.

They may never be able to do this competently in order to provide you with a road map to good eating and excellent health. They may find that it is easier to cure cancer than to find out exactly what causes it. We have already learned a similar lesson in curing many plant and animal diseases. When the plants and animals are fed adequately, with all known nutrients, the diseases go away; and that is cheaper and better than finding out exactly what is wrong.

In the meantime, while food scientists are studying these matters, we will struggle along with the knowledge and folk wisdom that have accumulated during the past 20,000 years.

One guide is that nature's assortments of nutrients in the tissues of staple foods tend to be biologically sound and

§ §

Dr. Linus Pauling questions guides for Vitamin C

One of the obstacles impeding the objective study of the role of ascorbic acid (vitamin C) in health and disease is that the amount of this nutrient we are said to need has been frozen by official edict. The very edict itself implies that we know how much vitamin C we need. In the United States, a recommended daily dietary allowance has been officially established by the Food & Nutrition Board of the National Academy of Sciences – National Research Council, an organization of distinguished scientists who look upon medical problems in the old, traditional way. . . . Thus, when it comes to establishing the amount of ascorbic acid (vitamin C) a person should ingest every day, they conclude that we need only 60 milligrams of this vital substance because this is thought to be enough to cure scurvy or to prevent it from developing. It turns out, interestingly enough, that this is the amount of vitamin C which is contained in the present diet of the average American. The Board has not made any serious effort to determine what daily intake of this vitamin would lead to the best health for the most people, to the greatest resistance to disease. This is certainly the wrong way to establish a daily requirement. . . . The British use the same strange method to arrive at their requirements. However, the corresponding British board has set the daily requirement at only 30 milligrams of vitamin C, which happens to be roughly the amount the people in Britain get in their food. . . . Now how can one explain the difference? We are no different in body constitution from the British. Our cellular structures are the same. . . . Thus, it is obvious that the British and U.S. authorities on nutrition cannot both

§ §

be right. The truth of the matter is they are both wrong. They are wrong because they both seem to have ignored the difficult question of how to achieve the best of health.

Let us examine man's evolutionary history to see what information it may provide about how much vitamin C we really need for optimum health.

Most animals manufacture ascorbic acid (vitamin C) within their bodies. Small animals have a lower rate of production and larger animals have a higher rate. The rate matches the body weight of the animal. The amount produced . . . varies between 2 and 15 grams a day for every 70 kilograms of animal. If we assume that no animal produces more of any substance than his body requires for full health, each of us requires not just 30 to 60 milligrams of vitamin C a day, but between 2,000 and 15,000 milligrams, that is, between 2 and 15 grams.

Consider the gorilla. He and we came from the same branch of the evolutionary tree. Like ourselves, the gorilla is a rarity among animals in that he has to obtain his vitamin C from his food. Unencumbered by knowledge of minimum daily requirements – there being no simian nutrition board – and with only natural food available to him in the jungle, the gorilla consumes about 4.6 grams of vitamin C in his diet of bamboo shoots and other vegetation each day. The average man, on the other hand, weighs somewhat less than half as much as the average gorilla, so if humans were similarly well fed, they would get 2 grams (2,000 milligrams) of vitamin C a day.

Dr. Linus Pauling. Reprinted with permission. "The New Medicine?" in *Nutrition Today*. September-October 1972.

make good eating and good health. This is not "going back to nature." It is only the utilization of good sense until a time when more reliable research information is available. We will, consequently, use this guide in exploring the whole foods that can be purchased in modern food stores.

FOODGRAM No. 2

Add sprouts to salads and health-building dishes

Are Your Salads Costing More and Feeding You Less?

Then add grain sprouts for low-cost vitamins, minerals, and proteins.

Seeds and grains are little storehouses of vital foods in balanced ratios. The seed skins are especially rich in vitamin B and food minerals. The germ portion has vitamins E, A, and D, plus protein and minerals in a good oil base. The seed core is a pablum of carbohydrates.

These nutrients explode into tasty forms when the seeds sprout and grow their tender shoots. The vitamin C of soybeans, for example, increases 500% by the third day of sprouting. The B and E vitamins also increase in value. Starch turns to sugar and the sprouts acquire interesting, zesty flavors.

Buying good sprouts is getting easier since people are shopping for them. Health food and Chinese markets usually offer them for sale. Some supermarkets have sprouts; others will soon follow as the demand is increasing. Many smart people are growing or buying seed sprouts.

In the meantime, until more stores sell sprouts, they are cheap and easy to grow in any house or apartment. (See Chapter 7 on Sprouts for additional information).

Here is a green salad recipe, with sprouts:

1 cucumber, sliced or cut to size
3 tomatoes, cut to salad size
Romaine or Boston lettuce
1 medium-sized onion, cut to size
1 cup of sprouts (alfalfa sprouts are good)
½ cup of salad croutons
French or Caesar dressing (or virgin oil salad dressing p. 61)

Mix and serve. The sprouts add over 40% to the vitamin and mineral values of this salad, plus contributing good protein.

Citrus fruits and juices have been popular foods for many years due to their good flavor and nutritional values, particularly in supplying vitamin C and food minerals. Rising food prices have stimulated a flood of imitation and diluted fruit juice products – for sale at lower prices. These sugared, flavored imitations cannot be accepted in an intelligent food shopping program. The whole fruits and juices are still the best buys for your money. If you need more vitamin C and minerals, they can be obtained as food supplements at health food counters and stores.

We compare the costs of vitamin C in different forms in this chapter and suggest breakfast beverages that will assist in getting essential supplies of this vital nutrient.

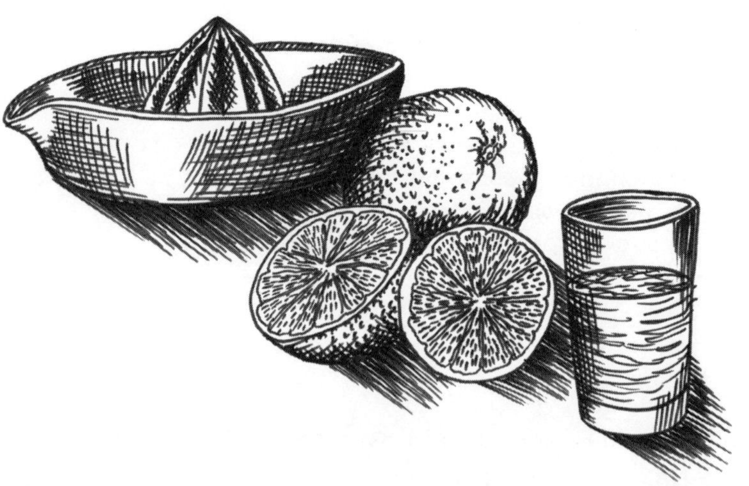

3

Oranges and Fruit Juices

Pasteurized orange juice is 53¢ a quart at our supermarket. Fresh oranges are 8¢ each, and it takes eleven of them to yield a quart of juice; so, home-squeezed orange juice costs 88¢ a quart – 35¢ more than the pasteurized product. Is the fresh juice worth the difference? Frankly, no one knows, but if you have a tight food budget even the pasteurized juice is a luxury.

Orange juice is offered in many forms in today's food markets: raw, pasteurized, reconstituted, frozen, and canned – and as an ingredient in imitation and diluted fruit juice products. These have many names, such as High C, Orange Drink, Awake, Help, citrus punch, fruit juice drink and imitation orange juice. One leading orange juice product shows the following list of ingredients:

> Water, sugar syrup, orange pulp, citric acid, cornstarch, cottonseed oil, potassium citrate, tricalcium phosphate, vitamin C, flavors, BHA preservative, sodium carboxymethylcellulose, coloring matter, and vitamins A and B.

What a departure from the citrus groves into the chemical factories!

The market appeal of these imitation fruit juices is low price. Some kinds of canned beverages are available for 35¢ per

History and kinds of citrus

Citrus is the Latin name for the *citron* tree. Linnaeus gave the name to plants belonging to the *Rutacae* family. Originating in Southeast Asia and Malaysia, the citruses were prized as fruits in China before the time of Christ. Alexander the Great carried them from Asia into Europe around 300 B.C., introducing the original small citron trees. Other varieties were brought from Asia to Africa and thence to Europe.

Columbus purchased orange, lemon, and citron seeds in the Canary Islands in 1493 and took them to America on his second voyage. By 1579, citrus growing was established in St. Augustine, Florida; by 1591, in Peru; and by 1769, Franciscan monks were growing citrus trees in California. The *wild lime* groves on the lower coastal keys of Florida were planted by Henry Perrine about 1838. Before his death in an Indian skirmish in 1840, he had established a nursery of over 200 species and varieties of useful tropical fruits, including citrus.

The valuable citrus family has many, many species:

Sweet oranges. Large, juicy, sweet fruits, including the popular Valencia and navel varieties.

Bitter and sour oranges. Grown to make marmalade and to provide rootstocks for other kinds of citrus trees.

Lemons. Unique acid-sweet fruits including Eureka, Lisbon, and Villa-France varieties.

Grapefruit. The distinct large fruit so important in American breakfasts.

Limes. The tasty, acid-sweet flavoring for drinks and foods.

Tangerines. Prized as a citrus specialty. Often eaten fresh or canned as a dessert fruit.

Kumquats. Grown in more northerly locations because of frost resistance. Prized in China, and often used for pickling and making conserves.

Clementine. A cross between tangerines and sweet oranges. Grown mainly in North Africa.

Chironja. A natural cross between Caribbean oranges and grapefruit. Makes a beautiful, tasty, tart-sweet fruit.

Tangelos. A cross between tangerines and grapefruit. Often found in food markets.

Ugli. A variety of tangelo.

Tangors. A cross between tangerines and sweet oranges. The popular Temple orange is a tangor.

In addition, limequats, orangequats, citranges, and many other varieties are grown locally for eating and taste specialties.

It is a rich and nutritious family of food plants.

46-ounce can, which equals 26¢ a quart – half as much as pasteurized orange juice and one-third as much as fresh juice.

Our task is to evaluate the various fruit beverages, find common denominators of value, and suggest the foods that may be acceptable in smartly run shopping baskets.

Why do people buy fruit juices?

People have been buying oranges, grapefruits, and citrus juices for many years, due to the vitamin C values of these foods and their good taste. Whole orange juice is, indeed, a nutritious food. It contains about 450 milligrams of vitamin C per quart of juice. Hence, an 8-ounce glass of juice has about 110 milli-

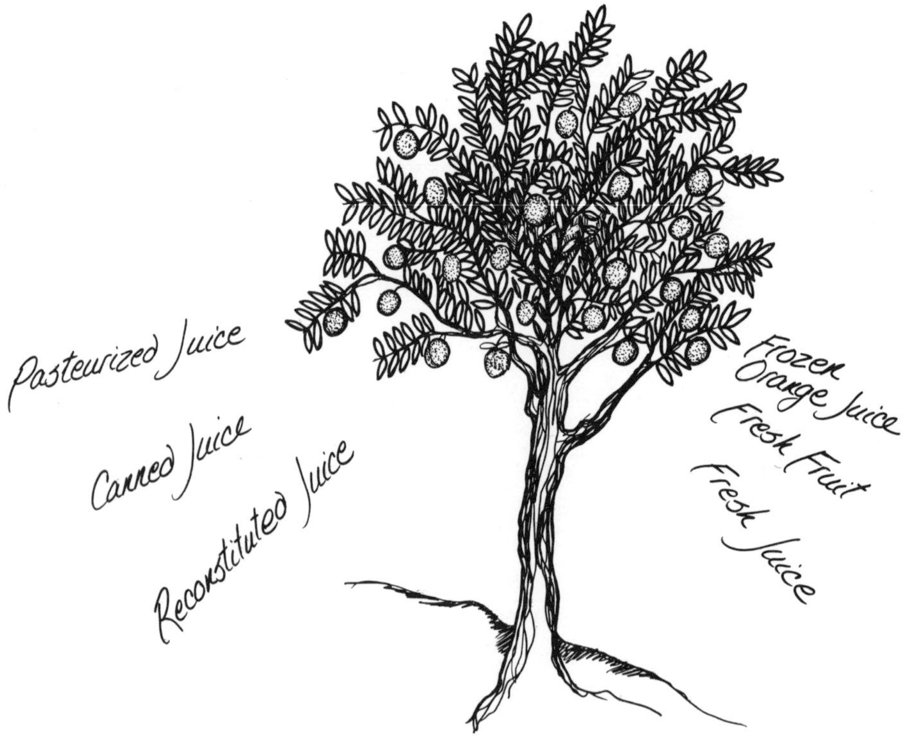

grams of vitamin C, and a 6-ounce glass (restaurant size) has 80 milligrams. Both of these quantities exceed the conservative Food and Drug Administration's recommended daily allowances (RDA's) of 60 milligrams a day.

Oranges are a whole food, however, and their vitamin C is intimately associated with many companion nutrients in the fruit. Whole orange juice contains significant amounts of thiamin, riboflavin, niacin, vitamin A, calcium, phosphorus, iron, potassium, and zinc as well as vitamin C, enzymes, and many other food fractions. These team together in providing vitamin and mineral nutrition – each nutrient improving the efficiency and values of the others.

This is called synergy (a good word to know), meaning that group action enables the individual nutrients to have an enhanced value because the others are present too. It is a way of making $2 + 2 = 6$, instead of just the old 4.

As an example, a subtle enzyme* in fresh orange juice protects the vitamin C from depreciation in the presence of air, helping the C factor to be more efficient.

In addition, citrus fruits and juices contain substances called bio-flavonoids, which are suspected of having valuable roles in human nutrition. It is a general term, and a number of food factors may be included; those presently noted in health food literature are rutin and hesperidin. One of the U.S. research leaders in studying this group of nutrients is Dr. Boris Sokoloff, at Florida Southern College, Lakeland, Florida. His studies indicate that vitamin C values in oranges and citrus foods are less than half of the total nutrient values, with the bio-flavonoid group being particularly effective in coping with diseases of middle and old age, including heart and circulatory ailments. This, however, is an underresearched field in U.S. foods and nutrition.

It would be a serious mistake, therefore, to count orange juice (or grapefruit juice) as a simple food, easily duplicated in food factories or replaced by concoctions of water, sugar, citric acid, ascorbic acid, color and flavoring agents.

Capable food shoppers have three values in mind when they buy orange juice:

¶ **Flavor and palatability,** so this food may add zest and pleasure to breakfast. Technically, this can be measured by a Brix test, which shows the sugar-acid ratio in the juice.

¶ **Vitamin values,** particularly vitamin C, but also including significant units of vitamins A and B. These values, too, can be measured by laboratory analysis.

* ascorbate reductase

Food mineral values, including calcium, magnesium, phosphate, iron, manganese, and zinc. The presence of these minerals also can be measured by simple laboratory tests.

Processing of orange and grapefruit juices

The oranges and grapefruits are harvested and hauled in large loads to the processing plants where the fruit is washed and pressed to expel the juice. A minimum of pulp is included since it contains "wild" enzymes that tend to make the whole batch unstable, causing "degradation."

The juice is then processed for four different kinds of products and markets: pasteurized whole juice, concentrated frozen juice, reconstituted juice, and canned juice. Typical processing operations are as follows.

Pasteurized whole juice is moved into a holding tank for 10 to 20 minutes and then deaerated (to remove air). It is pasteurized by flash heat at from 190° to 200° F to kill bacteria, enzyme, and other factors that would cause spoilage. The temperature is carefully controlled and does not rise above 200° F.

The pasteurized juice may then move to a bottling station for producing the bottled **pasteurized whole** juice to be bought in food stores. Or, it may move to a canning station where it is sealed in tin cans. The filling temperature, in either case, is about 188° to 190° F.

Canned citrus juice is simply the pasteurized product put into tins rather than into glass or cardboard containers.

Concentrated frozen juice may be subjected either to regular pasteurization taken from the pasteurized juice line, or it may be concentrated direct from fresh juice in an evaporator. In any event, the excess moisture is driven off by heat at a temperature of about 200° F. The concentration is to a quantity about 25 per cent of the original volume. Thus, in reconstituting such juice, you add three cans of water, remaking the full volume.

After concentration by heat, the juice is frozen and canned in the packages we buy in food markets.

Food values in orange juice

Freshly squeezed orange juice contains, per pound (about one pint), the following nutritional values:

	Milligrams per pound of juice
Calcium	50
Phosphorous	77
Potassium	907
Iron	1
Vitamin A	910 (International Units)
Vitamin B_1	.4
Vitamin B_2	.1
Niacin	1 .6
Vitamin C (ascorbic acid)	227 equals about 450 milligrams per quart of juice

Reconstituted bottled juice is the concentrated juice, watered to restore the original volume, and bottled or put into card-board cartons. It is usually labeled "from concentrate."

Vitamins don't act independently

It is a fallacy to imagine that vitamins and minerals act independently of each other, or of other foods. Some vitamins enable minerals to function; others enable the body to extract nutriment from certain foods, or are effective only when other vitamins are present. This is a general principle applicable to all the organs of the body, too, for if one organ is undernourished or fails, other organs become affected. Nutrition must be balanced so that the blood, which nourishes the whole body gets all the elements the body needs.

Harvey Day. *About Bread.*
London: Thorsons Publishers, Ltd., 1966.

Many studies have been made of the effects of these processing procedures on the vitamin C values in the products as compared with fresh juice. These studies show that the retention of vitamin C values is usually over 95 per cent even in the canned citrus juices.

The vitamin C value is evidently sustained quite well by processing. We do not know, however, what effects the heat treatments have on the many other food factors in whole, fresh citrus juice that may enhance the vitamin C value, and also provide added nutrition for people. Nutrition is a complex event of interacting foods. Research is still inadequate to give us clear-cut answers to many questions.

In the meantime, we must assume that whole, fresh citrus fruits and juices are the best products.

Vitamin cost in various products

The high prices of fruit and fruit juices have stimulated food suppliers to offer dozens of artificial and diluted fruit juice products for the market – usually as breakfast drinks. One of these, by some hook or crook, even got taken to the moon as a food for astronauts. They feature a vitamin C value and are offered at about 50% the price of pure fruit juices. One way to evaluate these imitation products is to compare them on the basis of vitamin C cost.

To do this, we can assume that half of the food value in pure orange juice is in vitamin C, and the other half in the minerals, vitamin A, bio-flavonoids, and other nutrients. For example, if a quart of fresh orange juice costs 88¢, then 44¢ is counted as vitamin C value, and the other 44¢ for other nutrients.

Here is a comparison of various vitamin C products, using such an approach:

Costs of vitamin C in various forms

Product	Net cost per quart ready to drink	Vitamin C value per quart	Cost per 100 milligrams vitamin C
Whole Orange Juice	.44	450 mgs.	10¢
Fresh	.44	450 mgs.	10¢
Pasteurized	.27	405 mgs.	7¢
Frozen (reconstituted)	.17	405 mgs.	4¢
Canned	.18	405 mgs.	4¢
A leading imitation juice	.22	240 mgs.	11¢
Another leading imitation	.24	unrated	?
Tomato Juice (canned)	.16	210	8¢
Vitamin C Pills			
"natural," from acerola base	$2.50 per 100 tablets of 100 mgs. each		3¢
Ascorbic acid pills	$.80 per 100 tablets of 100 milligrams each		1¢

This comparison shows:

- The pure juices offer more vitamin C for the money than the imitation and diluted products. At 11¢ per 100 milligrams of vitamin C, the imitation juices are the most expensive of all.

- Frozen and canned orange juice are good selections, offering more food value per dollar than the pasteurized juice.

- Canned tomato juice, also, is a good value for the money.

- Vitamin C pills, as a food supplement, are a much cheaper source of vitamin C – if that is all we are after.

- But straight ascorbic acid (synthetic vitamin C) is a still better choice from the cost standpoint – if all we are buying is vitamin C.

The food manufacturers are lacing their imitation and diluted fruit drinks with this low-cost form of vitamin C as a marketing appeal. Often, no other food value is provided or claimed, except sugar. The result is a "soda" rather than a food.

As this trend continues, we predict that many food shoppers will buy their vitamin C at the health food counters in the form of natural or synthetic vitamin C pills. By doing this, they may save enough money to afford real orange juice now and then.

The new food labeling guides

Soon, as you shop in the food markets, you will see new kinds of labels showing nutritional values in food and beverage products. An "imitation" orange juice label, for example, might look like this:

> ROCKET BRAND
>
> Imitation Orange Juice
>
> **Vitamin C-fortified**
>
> Each 6-fluid-ounce serving contains at least 6 milligrams of vitamin C (10% of adult recommended daily allowance).
>
> *Net 32 ounces*

Such labels are in keeping with the new food labeling regulations of the Food and Drug Administration, published in 1973. They say, in effect, that food products should have enough nutritional information on their labels so shoppers can make intelligent choices in selecting their purchases.

A summary of the new regulations for labeling imitation, diluted and fortified fruit juices is given on the opposite page.

Learn to read food labels!

This is one way to protect yourself and your pocketbook. The Federal regulations require food manufacturers to list major ingredients on the labels. The Food and Drug Administration regulation says:

> "Ingredients shall be listed by common and usual names in order of decreasing predominance."
>
> *(Section 1.10(h), Title 21, Code of Federal Regulations)*

§ §

Food labeling for imitation and diluted fruit juices and beverages

The new law says*:

A food shall be deemed to be an imitation, and thus subject to . . . the act if it is a substitute for and resembles another food but is nutritionally inferior to that food.

The word "imitation" must then be shown on the label.

No claim may be made that a food is a significant source of a nutrient unless that nutrient is present at a level equal to or in excess of 10% of the U.S. Recommended Daily Allowance in a serving (portion).

The new law also says that the label for a diluted orange beverage must state the percentage of orange juice in units of 5%, for example, 15%. If the amount is more than 0% but less than 5%, the label must say "less than 5%.

* Food and Drug Administration Regulations on Food Labeling, *Federal Register*, January 19, March 14, and August 2, 1973.

Therefore, when the label on a fruit drink says: "Ingredients: Water, sugar, orange concentrate, flavoring, citric acid, ascorbic acid and coloring" – then you know you are buying mainly water and sugar – and you have been **had!** This should be avoided.

Have your juice and vitamin pills

We do not see a future America of plastic people eating plastic foods, disregarding the pleasures of eating and the rewards of full lives. We see, rather, a future in which people will make sensible selections and compromises.

For example, a person may have his orange juice as a pleasant chaser for half a dozen food supplement pills. It makes sense because this provides assuredly adequate nutrition at lower cost and retains the zest of a tasty breakfast.

Taste and flavor, in the long run, are potent factors influencing what we eat. Vitamin pills have no flavor and

WHOLE FOODS FOR YOU

taking them is a bother. The flavors of artificial and diluted fruit drinks are scarcely better, however, and the vitamin pills are a better buy in foods.

The orange, prune, apple, cranberry, grape, and other fruit industries have learned to convert massive amounts of fruit tissues and juice into pasteurized, canned, and frozen products. Soon, these will have nutritional labeling so food shoppers can be informed about the nutrient contents.

An assessment of quality and value versus price indicates that these whole juice products are superior to the fab-

GUIDES AND SUGGESTIONS

Citrus and other fruit juices

Prices of fresh fruits and juices are already too high for many personal budgets. However, the diluted and imitation juices are no remedy – the actual food in them is very high priced. When the TV advertisement says, "Gee! This tastes better than orange juice," look out! Usually, you are being conned into buying colored sugar water and cheap vitamin C at a high price.

The following specific guides and suggestions may be helpful:

1. Include some fresh fruits and juices in your weekly diet, if possible. They probably contain nutritional values that are very hard to get in pasteurized, canned, concentrated, and frozen kinds.

2. Select frozen orange and grapefruit juice as a second choice. They usually have over 90% of their original vitamin C value, plus food minerals. They are basically good foods.

ricated, diluted, and imitation fruit drinks. They provide more vital nutrients per dollar of food shopping money.

Oranges and fruit juices

Some of these whole juice products are flawed, to be sure. Imperfect fruit may be utilized in making them; sometimes, they are by-products of other fruit processing operations. A great deal of pulp and solids, no doubt, goes into the pasteurized and frozen orange juice – perhaps some water too. These products are, nevertheless, beneficially influenced by the whole fruits whence they came. They are the best we can buy in most food markets short of the fresh fruit.

3. Also, choose canned citrus juices, tomato juice, and other whole fruit juices, to suit your taste.

4. Rely on the labels to determine whether they are pure fruit juices or imitations. The list of ingredients is the key. If it includes the words "water" and "sugar," it is an imitation or diluted fruit beverage and, usually, a poor buy.

5. If you need more vitamin C and the whole fruit products are too high priced, get some ascorbic acid (vitamin C) at a health food counter or drug store. It comes powdered and in crystals (granules) at about 20¢ an ounce (28 grams). It is harmless; people have been using it for many years in canning and jelly making. Use this cheap vitamin C and mix your own "high C" beverages. An example is given in Food-gram No. 3.

6. Choose vitamin C and mineral supplements at a health food counter or store to supplement your regular food diet – if you feel this need. The vitamin C complex is probably the best selection, since it usually contains the bio-flavonoids, derived from rose hips, acerola (Caribbean cherries), or other natural fruit sources. The cost of vitamin C in this form is still cheaper than in most other products.

FOODGRAM No. 3

Vitamin C fruit cocktail

Do oranges and other fruits cost too much, and do you want to get more low-cost Vitamin C?

Then, make a vitamin C fruit cocktail to add to your breakfast meal and for snacks.

This can be done by mixing vitamin C (ascorbic acid) into your regular orange juice or other fruit juice drink. The key idea is that the other nutrients in orange juice (or other fruit juice) will help your body to use this added supply of straight vitamin C. Working on this theory, it is best, of course, to use fresh, whole orange juice, since all of the "food companions" are in it, unmolested by heat and processing. However, the canned or frozen forms can also be used.

The straight vitamin C (ascorbic acid) crystals or powder can usually be purchased in 4-ounce (118 gram) packages for about $4.20.

The cost is then only about one-tenth as much as the cost of vitamin C in frozen citrus juice.

One level teaspoon of this added ascorbic acid contains about 4,400 milligrams of vitamin C.

The following recipe for a vitamin C fruit cocktail may be used as a guide:

1 12-oz. can of frozen orange juice (concentrated)
Juice of 2 fresh oranges to add fresh "food companions"
4 cans of water (instead of the usual 3 cans)
1 level teaspoon of ascorbic acid crystals (2,200 mgs.)
3 tablespoons of honey or other sweetener to balance the acid taste of the ascorbic acid. Use sugar, if you wish; it won't kill you.

Mix well. This makes about 2 quarts of breakfast drink.

Each 6 ounce glass of this vitamin C fruit cocktail contains about 250 milligrams of vitamin C. It's quality is fully equal to that in most vitamin C products sold in drug stores and health food markets.

The vitamin C in one glass is 4 times the FDA Recommended Allowance, and one-tenth the amount that Dr. Linus Pauling suggests as a daily intake.

Vitamin C is obtained, of course, in other foods you eat during the day, so this 250-milligram portion will serve as a solid unit of essential nutrition.

Raw oils and fats have been in the human diet long before history was ever recorded. They provide energy and flavor in foods as well as oil-soluble vitamins and fat compounds that are essential for vitality and resistance to degenerative diseases. Modern food oil refining removes many of these nutritive values, tending to leave a sterile, dead food. It is doubtful whether other parts of customary diets make up for this loss. Ways must, therefore, be found to restore the oil food nutrients in your personal diet and food selection program.

We describe, in this chapter, where salad and cooking oils come from and how they are made. You will find that these food oils come from seeds, grains, and nuts. If food processing removes vital nutrients from the oils, it becomes necessary to eat more whole seeds, grains, and nuts to restore adequate personal nutrition.

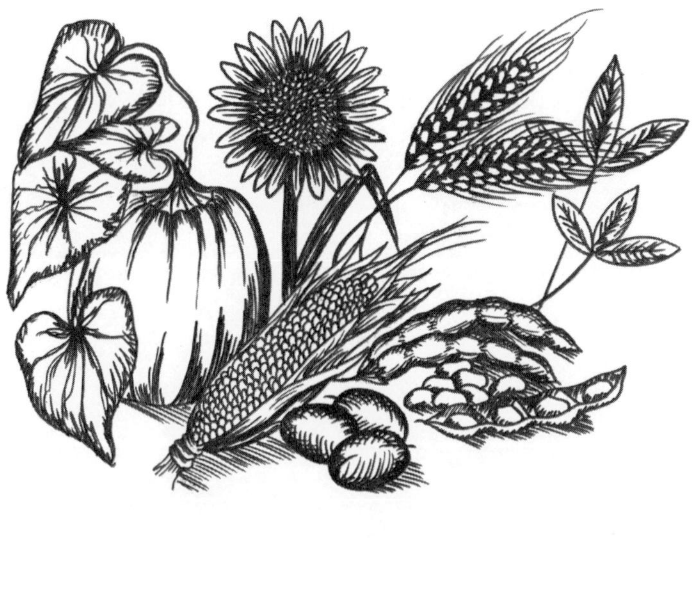

4

Food Oils

When an American housewife marks cooking oil on her shopping list, it is a fair bet that she thinks of it as a lubricant and frying agent, rather than as a food. Oil in the pan keeps meat and hot cakes from sticking. Hot oil makes french fries and "finger lickin' " chicken. Shortening in the dough makes tender crusts. Fat in the foods tastes good (sometimes) and makes them easy to swallow.

Lubrication and flavor, with nutrition as an incidental matter, have been the main roles of culinary oils in recent years. The oil food industry has responded by supplying beautiful, clear, odorless, tasteless, everlasting cooking lubricants – that may barely be classed as foods.

These attractive products are offered in supermarkets on the cooking oil shelves as various brands of corn, soy, peanut, safflower, cottonseed, and olive oils. The hardened (hydrogenated) vegetable oils are usually nearby in tins, fluffy white, for kitchen use. All of these products, with the exception of olive oil, have been extensively tampered with by men and machinery. Most of them have been subjected to heat in excess of 400° F. Their food values have been severely depreciated by the refining processes.

Many of the oils in health food stores also have lost

their original values. Cold-pressed types may have been heated to more than 300° F. in processing. Only a few suppliers produce lightly refined products. The truly excellent food oils on health food counters are those within the nuts, seeds, and cereals, still unharmed by modern industrial processing.

We make these comments not as natural food advocates in a now unnatural world but as food realists. We know where American cooking oils have been in their journey from seeds, grains, and nuts to the food stores, and then to your kitchens.

Fats and oils in human food chains

The oils in Earth's life systems are formed, initially, in the tissues of plants, particularly, in seeds, grains, and nuts. The germs of the seeds are especially rich in fats and oils. Corn plants, for example, store energy around the embryo (germ) of seeds for use by the new corn plants in their seedling stage of growth. These special tissues in the germs of corn seeds contain about 20% corn oil, whereas the whole seed has only 6%. The remainder of the plant has much less than 1%.

Other seeds may be richer in native vegetable oils. Walnuts contain 70% in their kernels. Wheat germs have about 15% in their tissues, while the entire whole wheat grain (depending on variety, area, and size of the species of wheat) may have from 1½% to 2½%.

Many vegetable fats that enter our food systems are found in seeds and nuts. However, some notable exceptions are olive, avocado, and palm oils where the fat is contained in the flesh of the fruits as well as in the seed kernels. Many plants also form tiny fat globules in their leaves and other tissues. Grass from fertile soils provides fats and oils to animals that eat it, and they, in turn, make fat meat and milk that we buy in food stores.

Human beings need fats and oils because we have eaten these foods since the very beginning of human history. We, too, cheek by jowl, ate leaves, seeds, grains, nuts, and fat fruits along with the other animals in prehistoric times. We then improved our eating skills and ate our fellow animals – birds, fish and insects – deriving vital oils and fats from them as well as directly from the plants, seeds, grains, and nuts.*

* Animals, including people, can also make some of their own fats from carbohydrates and proteins.

Our oil hunger is, therefore, about 4 million years old, at least. And we have depended upon certain oil-soluble nutrients over this entire span of time. Is it probable that our biological hunger would change much in the past 100 years – since 1874?

Our challenge is to obtain this vital nutrition at reasonable cost, even from today's food markets. An oil that is mainly a cooking lubricant and a deep-fat frying agent can hardly serve as such an essential food.

Food oils

The role of oil in our foods

Fats and oils have four principal roles in the human food systems:

- They provide heat and energy for our bodies.

- They add flavor and palatability to our foods. Think of a juicy steak, a sweet handful of nuts, or a slice of good bread and butter. The fats and oils provided much of the flavor.

- They supply essential fatty acids. These are oil-soluble nutrients, necessary for people's health.

- They provide the fat-soluble vitamins: A, D, E, and K, along with other soluble food factors such as octacosanols and phosphatides that assist in human hormone and metabolic activities.

Natural food oils and sex

It would be easy at this point to move into a description of natural food oils and vitamin E as key foods for sexual vigor and vitality. The oils and vitamin E concentrate in nature in the reproductive tissues of plants, and they clearly have a role in enhancing vitality of seeds and seedlings. Also, livestock breeders have known for many years that vitamin E and wheat germ oil improve the potency of breeding animals and sustain their vitality.

This is, however, an underresearched area. Adequate tests have not yet been made with human beings regarding specific values of raw food oils in sustaining vitality and a zest for life. We suspect that some of the eminent food scientists who deny the efficacy of raw food oils and vitamin E in sustaining virility and a keen interest in life might benefit from some surreptitious doses themselves.

In summary, fats and oils are wholly vital in human food systems. All of us must have these foods, especially the fatty acids and the fat-soluble vitamins A, D, E, and K in order to sustain health and to avoid an early onset of degenerative ailments and diseases.

Polyunsaturation —what is it?

The U.S. public has an amazing ability to learn big, complex words and ideas, particularly when product manufacturers and TV programs help them to do it. They know about spaceship modules, steel-belted tires, rotary motors, co-axial TV cables, radar scanners, and computer programming without having

---

Wheat germ oil and sex in animals

Bondonna and Kaan showed that wheat germ oil treatment to bulls resulted in a larger amount of semen of better quality and of greater viability.

Dukelow and Matalamaki reported an increase in number of lambs per one hundred ewes bred and per one hundred ewes lambing respectively.

Dukelow and Erickson reported that wheat germ oil produced greater numbers of spermatozoa in the second ejaculates in two of three experimental periods with bulls.

Aubel, Bay and Vogt-Moeller, Lentz, Crampton and Dukelow showed beneficial effects of wheat germ oil in the breeding performance of swine.

Farrell showed that experimental rats receiving octacosanol (a raw oil factor) required less time for reproduction and reflected higher conception rates than the controls.

Ezra Levin. Foreword to *The Physiological Effects of Wheat Germ Oil on Humans in Exercise.*
Thomas Kirk Cureton, Ph.D., Charles C. Thomas, Publishers. 1972.

Rancidity in fats and oils

Rancidity in cooking fats is caused by a chemical reaction between the fat and oxygen in the air, at the points in the chemical structures which are devoid of hydrogen. It follows that adding hydrogen to an unsaturated fat or oil will keep it from turning rancid. The fat or oil is then **hydrogenated**.

This process also causes the oil to become solidified at room temperatures.

In earlier days of American foods, the needs for hydrogenated fats were supplied mainly by lard from butcher shops and butter from creameries. With the rise of supermarketing, however, the food industry needed solid fats that were inherently cheap and would not go rancid – products with long shelf life at room temperatures.

The creamy, white, hydrogenated fats in tins, and oleomargarine, were the answers. These are regular cooking oils, hydrogenated for the solid fat markets and uses. They are unpolyunsaturated, if you please, by addition of hydrogen under high pressure and in the presence of heat.

If the theory of a cholesterol and polyunsaturated fat relationship is valid, these creamy, tinned, fat foods and most oleomargarine have lost their artery-protection values. They may be contributors to heart and circulatory diseases. Also, they have lost their vitamin E and essential fatty acids, if, indeed, any were left from the oil processing.

---

much chance to see what really exists and happens. In the case of polyunsaturated cooking oils in the supermarkets, it is still a deep, dark secret. What are these, anyway?

Polyunsaturated is an interesting plus-minus word, in any event. **Poly** means many. **Un** means without. And **saturated** means wet, soaked, or filled. How can you have many and still be without? What goes on here? Is this a food chemist's trick or a product-advertiser's gimmick? In fact, we are dealing with elementary food chemistry. Fats are compounds of glycerine combined with molecules of carbon and hydrogen, and of oxygen, called **fatty acids**. When the fats and oils possess – in their chemical structures – all of the hydrogen they can accommodate, they are called **saturated**. As units of hydrogen are removed, they become unsaturated. When more units are removed, they become polyunsaturated. That is the key idea. What does this have to do with the quality of a cooking fat or oil? Actually, not much, since the food values in the oil may have already been damaged by processing in any event.

According to existing research, the saturated oils (maximum hydrogen present) contribute most to cholesterol accumulations in human blood vessels. Unsaturated oils (medium hydrogen present) generate less cholesterol, and polyunsaturated oils (minimum amount of hydrogen) generate the least cholesterol. An accumulation of cholesterol in one's blood vessels is, of course, a contributor to heart and circulatory diseases.

Fats and oils are technically the same kinds of food compounds. The chemistry of each is generally the same, and the distinction between them is mainly one of hardness. Fats may be thought of as hardened oils.

Among the warm-blooded animals, each species constructs its characteristic kind of fat and the melting temperatures differ – the melted fats then becoming oils. Horse fat, for example, has a high melting temperature, about 150 °F. Pig fat has more oleic acid and is consequently, more edible since it melts at mouth temperature (about 96 °F). Beef and mutton tallow are a bit harder, needing higher temperatures before they melt. Milk fat and butter melt at mouth temperature. Pure butter is only an emulsion of butterfat and whey. When we bite it, it melts in our mouths.

An inquisitive biochemist is reported to have explored the effects of hard fats versus soft fats by feeding them to two dogs. First, he starved the dogs to get rid of their excess fats so they would replace it readily. He then fed one dog on sheep tallow, which melts at high temperatures, and the other animal on linseed oil, which is a supple fluid, never hardening at moderate temperatures. The poor dog with the sheep fat soon could hardly move, while the one fed on the linseed oil diet was limber as a weasel. The dogs, of course, recovered after a while by reforming dog fat from the abnormal fats that they had deposited in their bodies.

There is a lesson in this for people as well as for dogs: We do best on fats and oils with moderate and low melting points – and we should avoid hydrogenated fats. These, as a rule, are the creamy solid forms, sold in tins. They are made

What is your melting point?

Humans, without much furry protection, have relatively low melting points. The hairier mutton and sheep, with their warmer pelts, have harder fats.

We may notice the difference between various animal fats in our foods. In lamb dishes, for example, the fat solidifies even at mouth temperatures and may adhere to our lips and tongue. The fats of beef, pork, chicken, and butter have lower hardening temperatures and do not present this problem.

The hardening temperatures of a number of animal fats are as follows:

Animal Fat	Hardening Temperature
Mutton	101° (F)
Horse	100°
Beef	86°
Pork	82°
Chicken	75°
Butterfat	70°
Human	59°

from refined cooking oils, solidified by addition of units of hydrogen. Oleomargarine is a similar product, made from refined oils with color and flavoring added. The hydrogenated shortenings, which began their commercial existance as lard substitutes, have nearly displaced lard from food store shelves. In this process, some food values have also disappeared, along with the rich, distinctive lard taste.

Anticholesterols in raw food oils

There is mounting evidence that whole grains, seeds, nuts, and other vegetative tissues contain adequate supplies of nutrients to counterbalance cholesterol and avoid its harmful accumulation in human blood vessels. The virgin oils contain octacosanols, steroids, lecithins, phytopherols, tocopherols, and other nutrients that normally join with cholesterol in sustaining adequate human health. Present-day food processing strips these nutrients away from food oils and cereal products, with unknown and still unresearched effects on resistance to heart and other diseases.

These subtle companion food factors in virgin vegetable oils are greatly reduced and/or destroyed by oil refining processes. Dr. D. Kritchevsky* investigated the effects of heating raw vegetable oils to 392° F in animal feeding studies. He found that heating of the oil changed it sufficiently so that its inclusion in animal diets promoted the development of fatty plaque deposits in the blood vessels of the animals' hearts.

Clearly, the relations between food oils and human health and heart disease are underresearched fields, despite the fact that millions of dollars are being spent in preliminary studies. Life itself is a multiple-cluster thing, as are our foods. At some point, food and medical research must deal with clusters of nutrients together; if not, misleading information and poor guides will be provided for people wishing to improve their nutrition and personal health.

Until such research is conducted, we have no sensible alternative except to conclude that some whole seeds, grains, cereals, nuts, and lightly processed oils are essential in the diets of healthy people.

Dr. Wilfred E. Shute, a controversial and eminent physician, says:

> Historically, it is irrefutable that when new and more efficient milling methods were introduced into the manufacture of wheat flour, those methods permitting for the first time the complete stripping away of the highly perishable wheat germ, the diet of Western man lost its only significant source of vitamin E. Flour milling underwent this great change around the turn of the century, and it became general around 1910. The amount of vitamin E in the diet was greatly reduced, and with the loss of this natural antithrombin, coronary thrombosis appeared on the scene. . . . The result of the removal of our major, naturally occuring circulating antithrombin then explains our present day predicament quite fully.

Vitamin E for Ailing and Healthy Hearts,
by Wilfred E. Shute, M.D., with Harold J. Taub.
New York: Pyramid Books.1972, pp. 11–12.

* D. Kritchevsky and S. A. Tepper, *Journal of Atheroschlerosis,* 7:647 (1967).

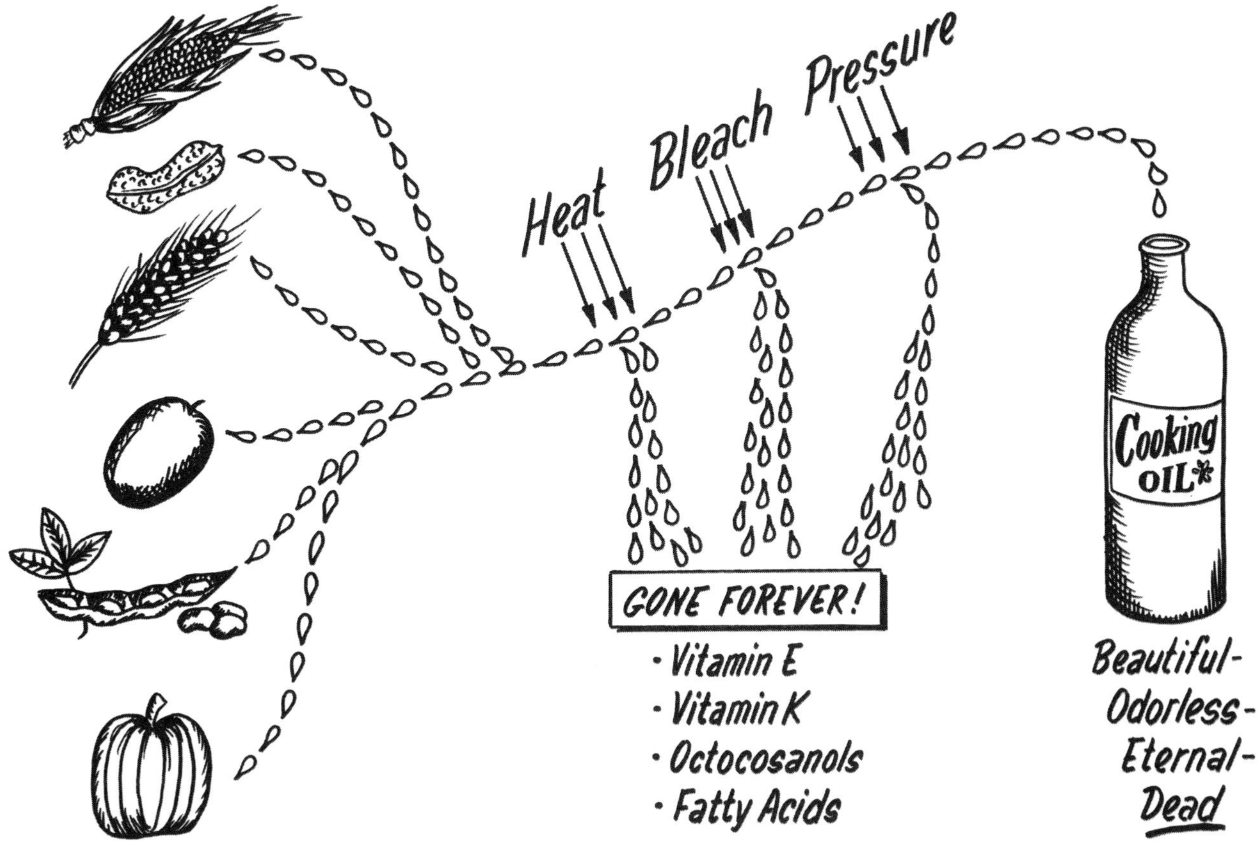

The beautiful, clear, odorless, everlasting food oils on the food market shelves have been treated, reacted, heated, flogged, reheated, washed, dried, and separated. These processes commit a rape of the virgin oils. Here is a nontechnical description of a typical food oil refining process.

Modern food oil processing

1. Extraction from Seeds. The seeds are rolled and heated to crack the cell walls and then are pressed to force out the crude oil. Temperatures are in the range of 300° F.

2. Treatment with Caustic Soda (Lye). Caustic soda (lye) is added to the crude oil in a process called treating. The lye reacts with free fatty acids in the oil to form soap. Insoluble in the oil, the soap settles to the bottom of the kettle and the neutral oil is siphoned off. Or, in high-speed continuous processing, the soap is removed from the oil by centrifugal force.

3. Drying the Oil. The oil is now heated to 220° F or more to remove moisture. The water escapes as steam.

4. Bleaching. Fuller's earth and charcoal are added, and the mixture is agitated for 20 – 30 minutes. These bleaching agents are then filtered off and the oil is put into storage for further processing.

5. Deodorizing. The oil is reheated to about 445° F and dropped down a series of plates in a column, where it is met by upward blasts of steam in a vacuum. The volatile fractions (odors) are carried up and away. The oil recovered at the bottom is essentially pure triglycerides.

This means, in layman's language, that the oil is nutritionally dead.

Food oil refining and soap-making

It is literally true that the refining of cooking oils entails a separation of the crude vegetable oil into an oil portion and a soap portion. One description is as follows:

The separation stage of the refining process is the most important as the results of proper pretreatment and centrifugation now become apparent. It is in the separation step that the yield of refined oil is determined. In continuous refining, high-speed centrifugals are used to separate the oil-reagent mixture into refined oil and soapstock. All of the previous processing has been in preparation for the separation stage.

Frank E. Sullivan. Lectures conducted by the American Oil Chemists' Society in *Refining of Oils and Fats* August 29–September 1, 1966, p. 87.

Admitting that this comingling of soap-making with food oil production may be objectionable from the aesthetic standpoint, it presents an even more difficult problem in nutrition. Substantial food values go into the soap and are forever lost to consumers.

Refined vegetable oils in the present-day U.S. food system have been so fully altered that their chief remaining value as a food is in energy calories. The bleaching process removes some of the phenolic compounds. Vitamin E is a phenolic compound that escapes in the presence of oxygen. Its value is surely reduced by the refining process. No one fully knows, or can state with certainty, whether refined cooking oils have effective vitamin E values that can be demonstrated by controlled testing, using real people as the testing universe.

Food oils

Does polyunsaturated, refined cooking oil help to prevent heart disease? No one knows. It is equally possible that refined cooking oils cause heart disease by removing vital nutrients from people's diets.

Herting and Drury* in work on tocopherals (vitamin E) in corn, wheat, oats, and rice compared the alpha tocopheral (vitamin E) content of these grains with the products made from them in food processing. They reported that "up to 90% of the Alpha tocopherol [vitamin E] was lost in the processing."

What is "cold pressed" oil?

The term **cold pressed** is an oddity of the food oil trades, usually meaning fairly hot processing, but not quite as hot as in the case of oil subjected to the full high-heat, deodorizing treatment. It is an oil that has been expelled from heated seeds or other oil materials, with use of substantial force and pressure. The temperature usually rises to 300° F to 325° F.

Adequate research has not yet been conducted to demonstrate the effects of this processing on food values in the oil. The heat and pressure probably destroy the chemical structures of the octacosanols and phosphatides as well as some other nutrients. Several superior food dealers will not handle oils labeled cold pressed unless the processing temperature has been kept below the boiling point of water, 212° F. This restraint would, theoretically, help to retain food values which could be destroyed by higher temperatures.

We reemphasize, however, that adequate research has not been conducted to determine the true food values of oils refined by various processes and at different temperatures.

* Dr. Hal T. Slover. "Tocopherols in Foods and Fats" in *Lipids*, Vol. 6, no. 5, 1971, pp. 291–296.

GUIDES AND SUGGESTIONS

Food oils and fats

There are two ways, we believe, that harm can be done to one's mental and physical health by poor quality food and bad food selections:

- To put toxic or harmful materials into our bodies, in excess of tolerable amounts, thereby causing illness.

- To omit essential nutrients in sufficient amounts, thereby causing malnutrition and an inability to resist illness and maintain health.

In the case of cooking oils, we doubt that these foods are toxic or that they may really harm you. They make good lubricants for frying pans and deep-fry baths for french fried foods – if you wish to eat french fried foods.

The problem is that these cooking oils are lifeless and fail to provide vital nutrients that have been essential in human eating systems for many centuries. Notably, the overrefined oils fail to supply fat-soluble vitamins and anticholesterol factors in our diets, although food oils have historically provided these critical nutrients and should continue to do so.

Where else can we get the vital oil-based nutrients for our personal use? Which food oils – if any – are acceptable?

The following suggestions may be helpful:

1. Use Mazola, Wesson Oil, Saffola, Crisco, and other leading oils freely as lubricants, but do not count on them as valuable foods.

2. Seek out in your market area, if possible, lightly processed food oils – and beware, those simply marked cold pressed, or cold processed – they may be little better than the major oils named above. Cold pressed is simply a trade term, and such an oil may have been heated above 250° and heavily processed.

3. A few lightly processed oils are available in some areas. The following have come to our attention:

Erewhon food oils, produced and distributed by Erewhon, Inc., Boston, Massachusetts.

Arrowhead brand, produced by Arrowhead Mills, Hereford, Texas.

Hain brand, produced by Hain Company, Los Angeles, But, only some of the Hain oils qualify. Look for those marked "unrefined" or "lightly processed."

Pure & Simple brand, produced by the Well Comany, near San Francisco.

Your action in seeking out such oils will encourage food store managers to stock them. Ask him to do so.

4. Select virgin olive oil for some of your needs, if you like it. But again, beware; some olive oils are getting heavily processed.

5. In any event, commence eating raw and lightly processed seeds, grains, cereals, and nuts – the original sources of good food oils. These are available as pumpkin, sunflower, sesame, and other seeds for eating as foods and snacks. The whole grains are available in whole grain breakfast cereals and in whole grain breads. Also, granola and familia are attractive seed, grain, and nut foods. Peanuts, peanut butter, walnuts, pecans, filberts, and almonds are good virgin oil foods.

6. Form the habit of eating sunflower and pumpkin seeds with your breakfast fruit juice. It is a good combination. And use seeds and granola for snacks.

7. For assured nutrition, supplement your diet from health food stores with vitamin E, wheat germ oil, vitamins A and D, lecithin, yeast, and other food supplements – to provide oil-soluble nutrients in your diet.

FOODGRAM No. 4

Almond-avocado virgin oil salad

Are your energy and zest for life a bit below par?
Do you wish to add raw food oils to your diet?
Then serve a virgin oil salad at least twice a week. It can be made of nuts, oily fruits, sprouts, wheat germ, sesame seeds, pumpkin seeds, and various kinds of salad leaves – to suit your taste.

Here is an attractive virgin oil salad recipe:

In a salad bowl, tear one head of green-leaf lettuce. Add two avocados, peeled, seeded and cut into ¾ inch cubes. Finely mince ¼ of a medium onion, with ¼ clove garlic and gently mix these into the avocado. Add 1 cup bean or other sprouts, if available. Gently toss all together. Garnish with 2 diced hard-boiled eggs and ½ cup of sliced or chopped almonds. Pour on enough virgin oil salad dressing to coat the ingredients (about 1 cup). Makes 4 portions.

The following recipe is suggested for the dressing:

Virgin oil salad dressing

In a blender put or blend with a or very fast whisk.

Lemon juice	⅓ cup
Honey	1 ½ tablespoons
Water	⅓ cup

Mix until honey is well dissolved. Add:

Dry mustard	1 teaspoon
Paprika	1 tablespoon
Salt	2 teaspoons
Cayenne pepper	⅛ teaspoon (1 whiff)

Mix well with the juices, honey, and water. Trickle in, while still mixing vigorously, 2 cups of virgin olive oil. Makes 3 cups. Use 1 cup for the salad and store the remainder. Blend again for use when needed.

Food Values:

Each portion of the salad, with dressing, provides:

Calories	600 (300 from dressing)	Thiamin (B_1)	26 milligrams
Protein	15 grams, high quality	Riboflavin (B_2)	.54 milligrams
Calcium	140 milligrams	Niacin	2.2 milligrams
Iron	4.6 milligrams	Vitamin C	24 milligrams
Vitamin A	1.535 I. U.		

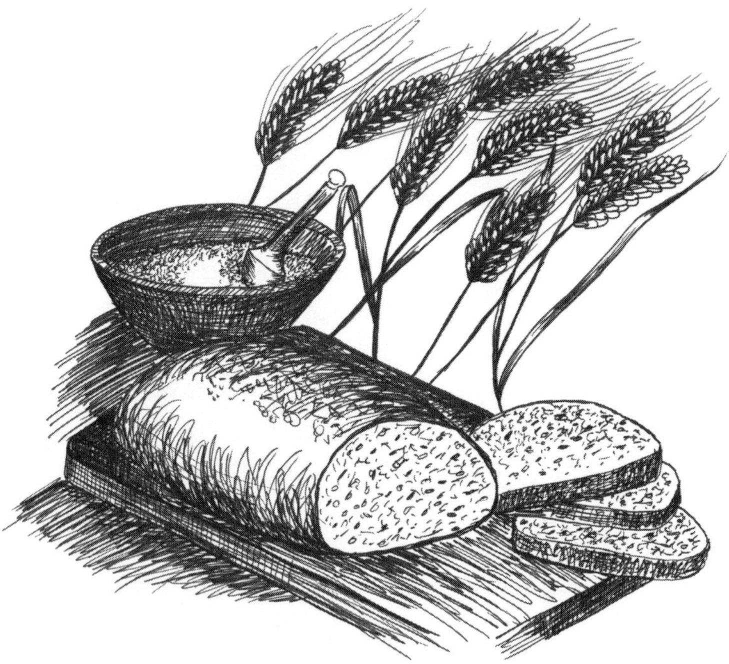

Whole grains are rich capsules of foods since they store all vital nutrients for new seedling plants. Ancient people discovered, many centuries ago, that the grains may also provide whole nutrition for us, and are good for bread-making. Wheat kernels have three parts: bran, germ, and endosperm. The starch and protein are mainly in the endosperm, vitamins and minerals in the bran and germs. Modern flour millers, intent on producing white flour, use only the endosperm, sending the bran and germs to the livestock feeders. This removes essential nutrients from U.S. food supplies. With rising meat, poultry, egg, milk, and fish prices, it is now necessary to restore wheat germs and bran to our foods. Making, buying, and eating whole grain breads are major steps in achieving this objective. In summary: Learn to buy and eat whole grain bread.

We describe, in this chapter, this ancient role of bread in people's lives. We describe the flour milling and bread-making processes, and show you how to get good bread again.

5

Wheat and Bread

Bread – our daily bread – give us this day – bread, the staff of life – he asked for bread and was given a stone. Of one thing we are sure: This was not wonder bread. Through all centuries until the present one, bread was equal to life itself in many regions of the world, because it was people's whole food. Once life was given, bread sustained it. Without bread, poor people perished; and most people were poor.

In America for the past 100 years, we have been able to switch from whole grain bread to white bread, having enough other nutritious foods to sustain us. Meats, milk, eggs, fish, and poultry have been fairly cheap and plentiful, and we have used them as providers of full proteins, vitamins, and food minerals in place of whole grain bread. Doing this, we could eat the billowy white bread as a luxury food – lovely but lifeless, and poor for the body.

However, the era is ending when white bread, meats, and diversified produce can serve as our national foods. Why? Because the meats, milk, fish, eggs, poultry, and fresh produce have become too expensive for most people to eat every day – in sufficient quantities for health and successful living. When good hamburger was 50¢ a pound, milk 25¢ a quart, and eggs 50¢ a dozen, people could eat enough of these good foods to compensate for eating poor bread. However, when meats and staple produce are priced beyond family food budgets, changes must be made or people will lose their health and productivity.

We are at that point in the United States; we have a dilemma: The traditional "protective" foods have risen too high in price for everyone to eat in sufficient amounts for health.

When hamburgers rise to 75¢ each in a land of hamburger eaters, and the meat is extended with various additives, fewer young people can eat hamburgers and the food value per burger declines. It may then become necessary to restore food values to the buns as a partial measure to sustain the health of young people.

The important point is that a large number of people will have to switch to whole grains and cereals – and nutritious bread – if they hope to sustain their health. Good bread will soon be an "in thing" in America. It will be useful to know and understand good bread when you see it.

Eating on the food chains

A web of life is a whole community of plants, insects, trees, birds, and other creatures in which each helps to sustain life in others. Big trees, for example, may fertilize succulent bushes with fallen leaves. The bushes, in turn, nourish deer and rabbits, which are eaten by coyotes; and fleas, ticks, and mosquitoes suck food from the deer, rabbits, and coyotes. Then each, in dying, fertilizes the big trees again.

The feeding part of such a system is called a food chain. It is an interlinking of foods, plants, and creatures in which each may nourish others in the same food system.

In the case of people, the age-old food chain is one where simple plants fertilize grass and bushes, which feed cows or buffalos, which, in turn, feed us. Then, we fertilize the grass and other plants with our wastes and contribute our bodies for the next grand cycle when we die.

We have steadily moved up on the food chain, especially in America, deriving more of our food from meats, fish, poultry, milk, eggs, and other sophisticated foods, instead of eating cereals and grains lower on the food chain.

Americans, for example, eat over 200 pounds of meat and poultry a year, per capita, compared with only 3 or 4

Wheat and bread through the ages

As a hunter turning toward agriculture, ancient man, over 15,000 years ago, probably used wheat and grains as food simply by chewing them. Then, as various civilizations developed, the grains were heated, eventually beaten, and mixed with water, and man ate his first grain bread. Today, wheat and bread provide more nourishments for people of the world than any other food.

Maza, which is a Greek name for a kind of porridge or paste, originated in Neolithic times. Wheat and barley pastes were quite common as bread. These pastes were flattened and heated or baked; and today, flatbreads exist as they must have been in Neolithic times. The Mexican tortilla, the Ethiopian injera, and the Indian chapati are offspring of the earliest bread of man.

Bread was the basic food for most of the early great civilizations – Egypt, Crete, Greece, and Rome. The upper classes ate as large a variety of breads as modern people do. By the Middle Ages, grain supplies in sufficient quantity were essential for the progress of the powerful countries. In Europe, wheat bread was considered the best of breads, fit for nobles. Barley bread became a staple food for commoners; and in the growth of Christianity and other religions, bread took its place among those foods sacred to hearts of humankind.

Cereal grains include rice, corn, wheat, oats, barley, rye, millet, and sorghum. Today, more than 70% of the world's croplands are devoted to production of these grains. Wheat accounts for the largest land area – 22%, and rice is second – 13%. Although rice supplies a larger proportion of total calories than wheat in the world's food, wheat is increasingly becoming more important because it contains – of all grains – more of the protein requirements needed by man.

For the above reasons, wheat is of vital concern to all people. If the richness of the natural grain is somehow lost by the time it reaches our tables and snack bars, it is important to know why, and more important to know what we can do about it.

pounds a year by the people of India and some other Asiatic countries. The East Indians could not possibly obtain even 50 pounds of meat for each person during a year. There is not enough to go around and it is too expensive. Consequently, they eat rice and other cereal foods direct, getting enough protein, minerals, and vitamins by eating lower on the food chain.

We need some good, low cost national foods in the United States. Something a man can bring home after work that doesn't cost too much and tastes good and is good for you, and that the family won't be mad about because it isn't a T-bone steak. Many countries and people have had good, low cost national foods – rice and fish, and whole bread and wine, sukiyaki, curried rice, tortillas and black beans, to mention a few.

What are our national foods? Cokes? Potato chips? Peanut butter sandwiches? Delmonico steaks? French fries? Man! We are nowhere!

Dick Gregory at Cellar Door,
Washington, D.C., 1972

We – Americans – are confronted with the need to do a similar thing: eat more seeds, cereals, and grains direct, rather than feeding them to livestock and poultry.

Frances Moore Lappe has described this situation in a beautiful little book entitled **Diet for a Small Planet.** We recommend it for a discussion of this phase of American foods.

Meat protein is permanently expensive

Only a few years ago (1940) 30 million Americans lived on farms, and meat was running around everywhere: cows, calves turkeys, chickens, sheep, pigs, pigeons, and rabbits out in the bushes. And in season, deer, pheasants, quail, and ducks were available. Meat had to be cheap because it was plentiful and nearby.

Knowing about foods

Suddenly I began to see the world's problems with food as my point of reference. Other facts began to strike me that I had previously taken for granted.

... I was amazed to learn that much of the critical study of plant protein is just now beginning to be done. For this reason, only now is it possible to leave behind the practically useless protein "guides" which purport to give the "amount" of protein in foods.

(I have had) tremendous personal satisfaction of being able to make real choices; indeed, how rare this is! Previously, when I went to a supermarket, I felt at the mercy of our advertising culture. My tastes were manipulated. And food, instead of being my most direct link with the nurturing earth, had become mere merchandise by which I fulfilled my role as a "good" consumer. But as I gained the understanding that I have tried to communicate to you ... I found that I was making choices, choices based on real knowledge about food and about the effect on the earth of different types of food production.

Frances Moore Lappe in Foreword
to *Diet for a Small Planet.*

Since then, our population has grown and America has been urbanized. Three-fourths of all the people live in towns and cities. This does two things:

- Eliminates farmers and the plentiful nearby meat supplies.

- Permanently raises the costs of growing, packing, refrigerating, shipping, and distributing meats – partly because they must be shipped farther and held longer on the way to market.

The end result, as we have seen recently, is to raise the price of meats in supermarkets to all-time high levels – too high for most Americans to afford everyday.

Beef, pork, mutton, and poultry are produced by feeding the animals and birds on grain, grass, and fodder. It was a good way to produce food in pioneer times when the livestock and grass were plentiful, but it is an expensive way to produce food when many people live in cities. About 5 pounds of grain are required to produce a pound of beef; 4 pounds to produce a pound of pork; and 3 pounds of feed to produce a pound of poultry.

Regarding protein itself, it takes about 8 pounds of cereal protein as feed to produce one pound of animal protein for us, as food. It is an expensive way to get good protein foods unless you live out in the country, own livestock, and have a big pasture.

Our challenge is to solve this food cost and supply problem in the supermarkets – within the United States food system in ways that are practical for everyday food shoppers and homemakers.

Good bread is part of the answer.

A Kernel of Wheat

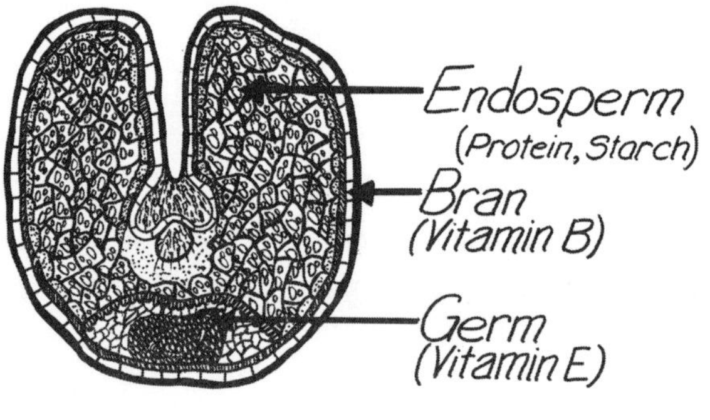

Grains of wheat Wheat, the breadmaker, is divided (like a good meal) into three parts:

❡ The Bran. This is the outer skin of the wheat grain, after the husk and chaff are removed. Made up of several layers, it can be removed layer by layer in milling to reach the white interior of the wheat kernel. The bran accounts for much of the brown color, flavor, and "chewiness" in whole wheat flour and bread.

The Germ. This is the live embryo, capable of producing another wheat plant. It lies at the bottom and side of the wheat grain, within a sheath which contains nearly 60% of the thiamin (vitamin B_1) of the entire kernel. The germ stores most of the oil-soluble nutrients for the new seedling and, therefore, is a source of vitamins E, A, D, and K.

The Endosperm. This is the creamy, white, starch supply in the wheat grain and also the main protein deposit. By careful milling, the food processors can remove the bran and germ to make pure white flour from the endosperm.

Wheat grains are so constructed that once the seeds have sprouted, the various parts of the kernels can provide complete, diversified nutrition to the new plants during their seedling stage. This helps to explain why whole wheat grains may serve as fairly complete human diets. When eaten whole, wheat provides balanced supplies of protein, carbohydrates, fats, and minerals, plus vitamin B complex and the oil-soluble vitamins E, A, D, and K.

True, wheat meal is deficient in lysine (protein unit) and several other special foods. Man has been making up these small deficiencies for ages by eating bits of meat, fish, eggs, fruits, nuts, and vegetables along with his whole meal bread.

The major foods in the parts of wheat are distributed in this fashion:

	In per cent			
	Bran	Germ	Endosperm	Total
Protein	19	8	73	100
Carbohydrates	7	4	89	100
Fats (Oils)	59	6	35	100
Food Minerals	77	.3	22	100

White bread is a starch and protein food. It was quite logical to become a favored food during our era of empire building and meat eating since the other foods provided essential vitamins and minerals, and meat was cheap. We now have a different situation, and must reconsider the food values in the bran and germs of wheat as well as in the starchy endosperm from which white bread is made.

An assessment of wheat grains shows that the major concentration of vitamins and minerals is in the bran and germ.

The distribution of the vitamin B factors indicates this concentration as follows:

	In per cent			
	Bran	Germ	Endosperm	Whole Wheat
Vitamin B Complex				
Thiamin (B_1)	13	64	3	100
Riboflavin (B_2)	42	26	32	100
Niacin	86	2	12	100
Pyridoxine (B_6)	73	21	6	100

A Kernel of Wheat, Chicago, Ill., Wheat Flour Institute.

As to food minerals, over 90% of these vital nutrients are in the bran and germ portions. The bran itself is rich in minerals as shown in the following table which compares whole wheat meal, unfortified white flour and bran:

In Milligrams Per 100 Grams, Dry Basis

Mineral	Whole Wheat Meal	White Flour	Bran
Calcium	51	20	118
Magnesium	157	30	565
Potassium	453	151	1265
Phosphorous	380	126	1305
Iron	5	1 ½	14
Zinc	4 ½	2	18
Manganese	4	1	12
Copper	1	Trace	1 ½

Kent-Jones and Amos. *Modern Cereal Chemistry*. London: Food Trade Press, Ltd. 1967, p. 35.

In summary, wheat has three parts: bran, germ, and the starchy endosperm from which we make white bread. This bread is fairly good for feeding loggers, high climbers, gandy dancers, bridge builders, ditch diggers, and farm hands – if they have enough other good foods. It is poor for people on 2,000 calories a day who sit down while they work.

Getting the wheat bran and germ back into the food supplies has become a No. 1 priority in America – more essential in the public interest than gas rationing or spaceships.

Victory or defeat?

Denmark had a critical food shortage in World War I, due to the Allied blockade of Germany. The country had 5,000,000 cattle and pigs and 3,500,000 people. The meager grain imports from America could not feed both livestock and people.

The government decided to slaughter 80% of the pigs and 16% of the cattle and give the grain they saved to the people. *All white bread, however, was banned.* The grain was made into whole meal. For the duration, the Danes ate whole grain bread, vegetables, potatoes, milk, butter, and fruit.

Quickly, Denmark was converted into a lacto-vegetarian nation. What happened? Many common illnesses nearly disappeared, and Denmark had its healthiest years. The death rate fell to 10.4 per 1,000, the lowest ever registered in Europe.

Harvey Day *About Bread* London: Thorson's Publishers, Ltd. 1966.

Making flour

Wheat is threshed in the fields with large combine harvesters and hauled to major flour mills, such as those of Pillsbury, General Mills, and Continental Grain Company. The grain is then milled into flour by means of the following processes:

1. Cleaning the grain. It is washed, cleaned, and scoured to remove all hulls, dirt, and foreign matter.

2. Breaking. The grain is passed through corrugated rollers to break it into coarse particles.

3. Removing the bran. The broken grain is sifted and treated with air currents to remove the bran layers from the rest of the wheat (germ and endosperm). The bran is used for livestock feeds.

4. Removing the germ. The flour is carried through germ rolls and sifters to take out the germ portions. The germ portions are used for livestock feeds and special markets.

5. Bleaching and conditioning. The off-white flour from these operations is bleached with chemicals to make it lily white for the elite American markets. Bleaching agents may include benzol peroxide, chlorine, chlorine dioxide, nitrosyl chloride, oxides of nitrogen, acetone peroxide, and azodicarbonimide.*

6. Enriching the flour. Selected minerals and vitamins are added to the devitalized white flour to restore a small measure of nutritional values. The usual additives of enrichment are thiamin (vitamin B_1), riboflavin (B_2), niacin, and iron.

The end result of these operations is a trouble-free flour: It will not spoil; bugs won't eat it; people buy it; bread bakers like it; and it is a very poor food.

Rate of extraction — what is white flour?

The white part of wheat grains – the endosperm – is about 80% of the whole kernals. The rest, too golden brown ever to become white, is discarded in making white flour and bread. Flour rolling mills unerringly find the line of separation, and this is stated in terms of per cents of "extraction," i.e., what percent of the grain was extracted to make the particular kind of flour? A 75% extraction, or less, can produce a white flour and bread. An extraction higher than 80% includes some bran and germ; thus, it cannot yield white flour and bread. The flour milling industry expresses this in the following words:

> Finally, flour extraction may be used descriptively to define a type of flour. Thus, if the proportion is 75% or less, a white flour is implied. If it exceeds 80% the flour will necessarily contain a significant proportion of non-endosperm particles. If the proportion approaches 100%, a whole-meal (whole-wheat) flour is being specified.
>
> From "Principles of Milling" in *Wheat Chemistry and Technology*, American Association of Cereal Chemists, St. Paul, Minn. 1971.

The end results of the various extraction rates on the nutritional values in the flour and bread are shown in the following table. It simply says: As more of the wheat grain is

* From list of permissible additives in *Wheat Chemistry and Technology*, American Association of Cereal Chemists. St. Paul, Minn., 1971.

Extraction Rate

	70% Pure White Flour	85% Mixed Brown Flour	100% Whole Wheat Flour
Total Minerals (ash)	.41%	.76%	1.55%
Oil (includes the oil-soluble vitamins)	1.17%	1.72%	2.52%
Thiamin mg.	.7	2.1	3.7
Riboflavin mg.	.7	.8	1.7
Niacin mg.	8.5	11.1	55.6
Potassium mgs/100 gr.	83.0	113.0	316.0
Magnesium mgs/100 gr.	27.2	45.1	143.0
Phosphorus mgs/100 gr.	98.0	141.0	350.0
Iron mgs/100 gr.	1.4	1.67	3.1
Zinc mgs/100 gr.	1.2	1.7	3.8

From "Principles of Milling." *Op. cit.*

used (higher extraction), nutrition goes up – dramatically, and in large amounts.

White flour and bread were developed originally for an elite market of wealthy people who could afford white bread as a luxury food – a status symbol. As political maturity was reached by working people and their wages rose in the past two centuries, they chose white bread to reaffirm the improvement in their social position. Also, they acquired a taste for it.

Flour millers and bakers have encouraged this trend since it is cheaper to make and sell white bread than the more nutritious whole grain kinds.

Making american white bread

America bread bakers used the time-honored sponge and dough methods – mixing, kneading, rising, and baking – until the 1950's. Some ingenious bread men then demonstrated that intense mixing and beating could replace the traditional fermentation with yeast, blowing up and pumping air into the dough. They also learned how to pump and extrude the dough, saving a great deal of time and hand labor.

These high-speed innovations, called "continuous breadmaking," were adopted in the United States bread industry during 1950–1970; and they prevail today. Old-fashioned bakers who use the slower methods make a superior loaf of bread, but they cannot compete cost and pricewise with the "beat and pump" bread factories.

Here are the steps in continuous breadmaking:

1. **Making the ferment.** A broth is made of yeast, sugar, milk, salt, enrichment, and mold-inhibitor (sometimes some flour).

2. **Mixing the dough.** The ferment is blended with the mass of dough, which is then sent to a pumping vat unit.

3. **Developing the dough.** The pump delivers the dough into a "developer" which beats and mixes it with intense energy for a few minutes, removing the need to "raise the dough" with the time-consuming "sponge" process.

4. **Extruding the dough.** It is extruded under pressure into baking pans.

5. **Baking.** The bread is carried on endless belts through the ovens while it is baked.

The end product of this continuous breadmaking process is the billowy, soft, white bread on the supermarket shelves.

When bread advertisers show those soft loaves on TV, dancing as delighted old ladies squeeze them in supermarkets, it is only their effort to help you to accept this arid food.

Whole grain flour, full of texture and life, is difficult to use in high-speed breadmaking. It defies dead-level chemical and mechanical processes that save 100% of human effort. At present, the conventional sponge and dough methods are essential in making whole grain breads. Also, good flavor in bread is generated by the slower marriage of yeast, grain, milk, and other ingredients.

Pepperidge Farms and other good breadmakers report that the demand for good whole grain bread is rising. The costs can be lowered as the volume of demand increases.

Continuous breadmaking

Continuous breadmaking in comparison with conventional methods, reduces processing time, and floor space, and saves labor.

Much controversy has centered about consumer acceptability of continuous bread. A typical slice of continuous bread possesses a very fine, uniform grain structure and a crumb that is soft and lacking in strength and resilience; continuous bread is often said to be "cake-like" and to lack flavor. This type of bread has been accepted in many markets but has encountered resistance in others.

"Continuous Breadmaking" in *Wheat Chemistry and Technology*, American Association of Cereal Chemists. St. Paul, Minn. 1971.

Margaret Rudkin of Pepperidge Farm

One day in the 1930s Margaret Rudkin of Pepperidge Farm found an old recipe by her grandmother for 100% whole meal bread. She used honey as the sweetener to make the yeast work.

Margaret ground wheat in the coffee grinder and made her first loaf of bread – firm, tasty and good to eat. She offered it to her friends and neighbors and they demanded more. Soon she was making and selling the first Pepperidge Farm bread.

Today, Pepperidge bread is sold in more than 100,000 stores as an elite white bread, but also as whole grain loaves in the original tradition of good foods – good breads. The company now offers over 20 different kinds of bread.

A 100% whole wheat bread has a shorter shelf life – it spoils quicker because it is alive and nutritious. The new sprouted grain breads help to overcome this problem. They are popular and have a good future. The sprouts, having exploded some units of energy, are stable in the bread and very nutritious. Buying these loaves helps good bakers to stay in business.

Is enriched bread a whole food again?

Life on earth is sustained by pairs, groups, clusters, and whole constellations of nutrients interacting and working together – never by single foods. In the case of simple forms of life, the variety may be less essential for example, in adequately feeding a lichen or a diatom. They at least do not need critical supplies of vitamin B to nourish brain cells.

In the case of people, the process of feeding is wonderously complex. At least 40 different food minerals may participate in feeding you, and no one will ever know exactly how they affect each other – and you.

Then, add dozens of vitamins, fatty acids, amino acids, carbohydrates, and enzymes to the list. Relate them to the 40 food minerals and you begin to understand about human nutrition – and the enrichment of bread. Real richness is amazingly complex.

Also, you understand the importance of whole foods – kinds where you can obtain whole clusters of nutrients at one healthy bite or in one tasty meal. Most people do not care about which mineral is being eaten and what catalysts helped it to provide nourishment, as long as life is sustained.

With such a preface, we can think validly about enriched bread. We know that the wheat grain was raped in milling. About 90% of its nutrients were stripped away, leaving mainly starch and protein. At least 100 different nutrients were removed from the scene, and no matter what might be restored via enrichment, the clusters are broken. Normal interactions and catalytic effects among the different nutrients are no longer possible.

The enrichment of white bread is performed by bread bakers under the regulations of the Food and Drug Administration. At present, specific amounts of thiamine (B_1), riboflavin (B_2), niacin, and iron (Fe) are authorized by FDA. Their addition to white bread is commendable as an effort to prevent pellagra, anemia, and other deficiency diseases but does little to restore full nutritional value.

Wheat and bread

The Food and Drug Administration has recently approved the iron enrichment to 25 milligrams per pound of bread, which approximately doubles the amount added over the previous level. This, it is said, will help to overcome iron-deficiency anemia which is found to be prevalent in the United States.

Again, this increase may be commendable, partially to restore one of the many nutrients that has been removed from bread by bad milling practices.

It is time, however, for a different perspective. Iron-deficiency anemia is only an indicator of an across-the-board deficiency of many nutrients in the diets of Americans. Iron is always linked with manganese, copper, zinc, and a dozen other nutrients in feeding both plants and people. If we need more iron in our bread, we probably need manganese, zinc, and other minerals too.

If we need thiamin, riboflavin, and niacin, we probably need their food companions (dozens of them) and also more of vitamins E, A, D, and K – that were discarded in the wheat germs.

There is only one adequate answer as far as bread is concerned: Buy whole grain bread. Wheat, rye, or any mixture – select whole grain bread.

Graham, Roman meal brown, and special breads

The bread shelves are filled with special kinds of bread that appeal to mild health food customers and people with a liking for brown bread flavor. These may be selected for personal taste and to break the monotony of eating (if you need that) but they should not be expected to equal whole grain breads in nutritive values.

Graham bread contains some unsifted whole grain flour. It also may contain, mainly, white flour. Examine the list of ingredients. It will tell you what kind of flour predominates.

Cracked wheat bread is just that. It contains cracked wheat, but often you cannot tell whether it is cracked whole wheat.

Pumpernickel bread is made from rye meal. If this is the principal flour ingredient, it can be an excellent bread.

Bagel is an interesting bread that is boiled before being baked. The ingredients are usually superior, and bagels may be from different kinds of flour – white, whole wheat, or mixed.

Commercial "wheat" bread is simply a modified white bread, with some whole wheat flour added. It offers limited nutrient values.

§ §

Learn to read bread labels
it is as fascinating as mystery stories

Remember, Federal law requires the breadmakers to list the main ingredients, "by their common names, in order of decreasing predominance" (Section 1.10(h), Title 21, Code of Federal Regulations).

To illustrate, let us take a poor quality bread.

First, one that claims that it "helps build strong bodies 12 ways."* It is "made with enriched flour, water, corn sweetener, shortening, yeast, salt, soy flour, whey solids, dough conditioners, yeast nutrients and calcium proprionate (a preservative.)" Such a label reveals that the soy flour portion is less than the salt portion, making the soy flour portion quite small.

Second, let us examine the label of a medium-quality, mass-production bread, called a "wheat" bread. Its list of ingredients says, "Flour, water, whole wheat flour, corn syrup, liquid sugar, shortening, yeast, salt yeast nutrients and dough conditioners, caramel color, malted wheat flour." In this case, whole wheat flour is a noteworthy ingredient, although less than white flour. Caramel coloring accounts for the golden brown color, and the malted wheat flour must be of very small amount, since it is less than the salt in the loaf.

* Registered trademark.

Soy bread contains, of course, soybean meal. The label will indicate, however, what other kinds of flour are included.

In summary, there are many kinds of bread – and good kinds not listed here. Societies seem to show their complexity and values by the kinds of breads they eat. But traditionally, poor people overcome and inherit the earth – possibly because, in the due course of events, they eat coarse, whole grain bread.

§ §

Third, a commercial grade, 100% whole wheat bread. Its statement of ingredients says, "Stone ground whole wheat flour, water, molasses, liquid vegetable shortening, corn syrup, non-fat dry milk, yeast, salt, dough conditioner." This is probably a good bread. Notice that it contains milk and molasses, and that the amount of dry milk at least exceeds the salt. If the first bread above can help build strong bodies 12 ways, this one should be able to do it in at least 24 ways.

Fourth, a commercial sprouted wheat bread. It contains, according to the label, "100% whole wheat flour, water, sprouted wheat kernels, sesame seeds, raw wheat germ, sun dried sunflower seeds, honey, soybean oil, salt, brown sugar, unsulphured molasses, fresh yeast, vinegar and lemon juice." What a symphony! How many ways can it build strong bodies?

Fifth and finally, a very dark "black" bread. The label says it contains, "Flour, water, rye flour, dextrose yeast, caraway seed, shortening, salt, wheat gluten, caramel color, yeast nutrients, and dough conditioners." It is typical of many breads in the markets made mainly of white flour and colored dark brown to simulate a whole grain bread. We believe this bread is nutritionally similar to the wheat bread listed as secondly above.

Read the bread labels, and select foods with your eyes open.

GUIDES AND SUGGESTIONS

Wheat and bread

The personal guide is clear: Select and eat whole grain bread. Use the list of ingredients on the label to decide which loaves are worth buying.

Suggestions for improving bread supplies in your neighborhood – where you shop – are more complex. Some stores do not carry whole grain breads, and it is a task to get the manager to stock these vital foods.

1. If your store does not offer good bread, talk to the manager. Ask him to provide it, and tell him why.

2. If several of your friends and neighbors wish whole grain bread, too, get them to join with you in visiting the store manager.

3. Check on the kind of bread used in the school lunch program – if you have children. If they are not serving whole grain bread, at least as a choice on some of the lunches, request that they do so. And again, see if your neighbors will help to get good bread into the school lunches.

FOODGRAM No. 5

Wheat and cheese together

Do You Need Another Way to Beat High Meat Prices?

Then eat whole wheat bread and cheese together. The combination raises their protein value by 25% and gives many of the vitamin and mineral values of good red meat.

Here is the analysis:

A.	Eaten separately:	In Protein Value
	1 ounce of cheese equals	1 ounce of steak
	4 slices of whole wheat bread equals	1 ounce of steak
	Total	2 ounces of steak

B. Eaten together:

1 ounce of cheese plus 4 slices of whole wheat bread equals	2½ ounces of steak
Increase	25%

Again, the amino acids in the cheese and wheat fit together to make a high-quality protein "bite."

Toasted cheese sandwiches make a good combination of these foods. They are easy to make:

butter the bread lightly on the outside of the sandwich.

Put the cheese slices inside.

Heat up the electric frying pan, or any other suitable pan.

Toast your sandwiches on each side.

Some readers may wish to start making homemade bread. We offer the following recipe for their use:

MAUDELLA'S WHOLE WHEAT BREAD

This bread recipe was developed during World War II to assure good nutrition, even though some foods were in short supply. Our old friend, Maudella (Mud) Vincent, took it to the Olympic Peninsula, Washington, used it for years, and shared it with neighbors. It has a fine flavor.

RECIPE FOR FOUR LOAVES OF BREAD

2 packages yeast (active or dry)
2 eggs
¾ cup honey
1 quart milk
4 tablespoons oil or melted butter
4 teaspoons salt
4 pounds flour (whole wheat)

Mix yeast in large bowl (moisten first if using dry yeast), pour in honey and salt, mix, set aside until it foams. Mix in eggs and oil, stir well. Gradually mix in heated milk (not too hot), stir well. Sift in flour. Stir in liquid mixture gradually until too stiff to stir. Empty onto floured bread board or flat surface. Put more flour in until mixture is thick enough to knead. Knead it well (about 5 minutes) until a little sticky. Put dough aside in warm spot and let it rise until it has doubled its size (takes about one hour). Punch it down and form into loaves. Put loaves into greased bread pans and let rise until again about doubled. Bake in 325° to 350° oven for 1 hour.

Americans ate nutritious breakfasts for 250 years, usually including cooked cereals in one form or another. With the rise of TV advertising and high-speed living, our breakfasts have changed, notably by eliminating cooked foods and substituting dry and sugared cereals. Nutritional analysis shows that even the best of these are mediocre foods at high prices. The sugared kinds are atrocious at any price – confections masquerading as foods for children. Eating whole seeds, grains, and nuts for breakfast – along with fruit juices – is one of your *alternatives in choosing better foods. Sunflower, pumpkin, and sesame seeds are good selections, with granola and familia as palatable forms of these nutritious foods. Guides and recipes are given.*

We describe in this chapter the bad trends in breakfast foods in recent years, and suggest the choices you can make of good cereal foods for this important meal.

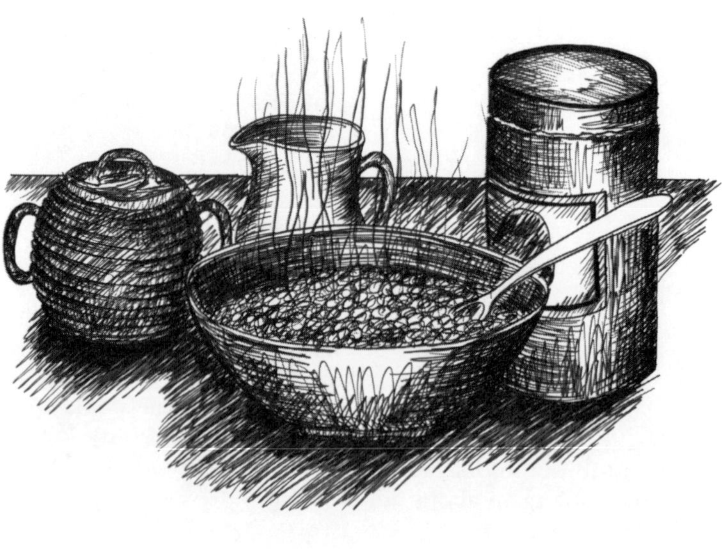

6

The True Values of Breakfast Cereals

We may speculate: What did cave people eat for breakfast before going out to hunt for rabbits, lizards, and mountain hens?

Many times, no doubt, they went hungry, but we think the smart cavemen – who emerged as our ancestors – ate seeds and nuts for breakfast, thereby having good spirits and sharp eyes for the day's hunting. Why not? The seeds and nuts could be gathered and stored; a handful made a nutritious meal. And they taste good. Good foods have been "sweet as a nut" ever since morning-time in human history.

Traditional American breakfasts for 250 years nearly always included grains and cereals in one form or another. The Quakers ate oat porridge, later called oatmeal mush. It became the morning food for millions of farmers, tradesmen, and working people. Oatmeal performed well as a staple food, since a handful provided 14 grams of protein, 7 grams of food oil, 300 calories of energy, 2 grams of food minerals, and an assortment of vitamins. The protein, oils, and minerals in a bowl of oatmeal mush were one-fourth of a day's needs – just right for a good breakfast when eaten with eggs and a bit of meat.

The Quakers and other early Americans felt this nutrition and found that it was good, rather than counting the grams, milligrams, calories, and International Units (I.U.). The counting came later, as breakfast foods declined in nutritional values.

Corn was a main breakfast food in other parts of America. Corn porridge, bread, grits, and hominy fed planters, slaves, tradesmen, workers, and sharecroppers alike during 250 years of Southern life. The early laws in some states required planters to provide at least 20 pounds of corn meal and 3 pounds of pork a week to each of their farm workers (slaves).

One pound of whole corn meal provided 42 grams of protein, 18 grams of food oil, 1600 calories of energy, 5 grams of food minerals, and a cafeteria of vitamins. When eaten with pork and a bit of greens, it became whole food for hard-working people. Eaten for breakfast, it kept stomachs from rubbing backbones until noon.

Both oats and corn are **cereals** – the fruits of **grasses.** They are seed parts which – like wheat – contain whole clusters of vital foods capable of acting in concert, with each nutrient improving the contributions of the others. Barley, millet, sesame, rice, and rye have similar nutritional powers.

The decline and fall of American breakfasts

Half rural and too active to get along on "empty" foods, Americans sustained the integrity of their breakfasts fairly well until 1950. Cooked cereals, corn flakes, milk, ham and eggs, bacon, toast, muffins, biscuits, butter, grits, hashed browns, hot cakes, corn bread, sausages, and cocoa and coffee were our staple breakfast foods. None of these needed expensive Madison Avenue promotions in order to be sold.

Two powerful forces have changed this earlier breakfast system: TV advertising and the urbanization of America – the movement of many people out of rural America into the towns and cities – into supermarket country.

TV advertising taught 50 million children and young people to eat sugared and heavily processed dry breakfast cereals—taught them for life, and switched millions of mothers and daddies into eating the same quick, convenient meals.

In 1940, only six dry cereals were offered in most food markets: corn flakes, bran flakes, shredded wheat, grape nuts, puffed wheat, and rice crispies. Five feet of shelf space in the food store was enough for selling these foods. Today, many supermarkets offer 60 different kinds of breakfast cereals from Kaboom to Sugar Smacks via Bran Buds, Fruit Loops, Apple Jacks, Clackers, Stars, Lucky Charms, Twinkles, Sugar Jets, FrostyO's,SugarPops,Kix,Trix,CaptainCrunch,CrispyCritters, Krinkles and Frosted Flakes – taking about 50 feet of three-deck display space, or a total of 150 linear feet to offer these highly advertisedfoods.

The true values of breakfast cereals

Old-fashioned cooked cereal breakfasts have virtually disappeared from American homes in the past 25 years and have replaced by dry cereals and other quick breakfast foods – or by the morning snack after getting to work or school.

The U.S. Department of Agriculture surveys of family food consumption, although not up to date in measuring these trends, show:

Average pounds per family per week *

	In 1942	In 1965
Dry ready-to-eat cereals	.4 lbs.	.8 lbs.
Cooked cereals	.8 lbs.	.3 lbs.

*Data from Food Consumption Group, Agricultural Research Service, USDA.

We suspect that these trends toward dry cereal breakfasts have been accelerated since 1965, with the result that dry cereals are staple breakfast foods for over 80% of all Americans, insofar as they eat breakfast meals at all.

TV advertising, beamed at children, served as a powerful force, accountable for this drastic change in American breakfasts in the past 30 years.

The advertising blitz

TV advertising on children's programs is the major force causing the deterioration of breakfasts. Urbanization put people into large mass-buying groups, capable of supporting supermarkets; TV advertising told the children what to eat for breakfast. The children told their mammas, and sugar-frosted

Quaker oats

In the 1850's, American breakfasts often took about two hours to eat. European visitors were revolted by the huge meals, consisting of salt fish, beefsteak, sausages, boiled fowl, ham and bacon, together with corn bread in gravy, jam and honey, potatoes and other vegetables.

Oats as food was not very popular. Scotland was considered the home of oats or oat porridge. In fact, eating oat cereals by humans was considered insane and inappropriate by most people in society. Newspapers chided oat eaters as robbers of horses, and said that oat eaters would develop whinnies, and horses' diseases as well. In fact, most oats were imported from Scotland or Germany for American consumption [which was not large].

Ferdinand Schumacher, a German immigrant, was quite a loner when in 1854 he rigged up a hand mill for grinding oats in the back room of his little grocery store. "The general opinion prevailed" he wrote later, "that our domestic oats were not suitable for the manufacture of oatmeal. After satisfying myself that this was a mistake, I laid the foundation on a small scale of my present extensive milling establishments – and became the pioneer oatmeal manufacturer."

The location of the little "oat king" mill was in Akron, Ohio. The Schumacher oatmeal was a cheap protein, not only for breakfast, but as a meat substitute at any meal. German migrants heard about the Akron Avena mill from their Cleveland compatriots. Not long after this, oats were being shipped in glass jars to New York and Philadelphia. And outgrowing both grocery and hand mill, Schumacher in 1856 organized the German Mills American Oatmeal Factory. He used a waterwheel for power, and between stones, he would daily grind enough oatmeal to fill 20 180-pound barrels. At first oats sold in bulk, then in jars.

In 1873, the first standard American cookbook to contain a recipe for oatmeal [except as a sickroom gruel] appeared – with a formula for oatmeal mush. In 1877, the Quaker Mill Symbol was given commercial form – when the figure of a man in Quaker garb was registered as a trademark. This was America's first trademark as a breakfast cereal.

In 1886, Ferdinand Schumacher had just filled his bins with 100,000 bushels of oats, plus a supply of other grains. He owned the largest oat milling complex in the world. His Jumbo Mill, only 3 years old, was five stories high and a mechanical wonder. He had introduced to America the use of oatmeal as a human food, and had created both an industry and a staple substitute for meat. Schumacher was the largest employer, the heaviest buyer and the biggest industrialist in Akron. The economy of the area had grown up around him. So when his mills burned down in 1886, everyone was affected. The immigrant miller watched his life work burn up. When asked why he wasn't insured, he said: "They want a fearful price for premiums; I wouldn't pay," he replied in heavy German-accented English.

After the great oat mill fire, Robert Stuart, from a small mill at Ravenna, Ohio, 16 miles from Akron, began selling oats under the Quaker package which displayed a lean austere Quaker. Stuart, Henry Parsons Crowell, and Schumacher can be considered as the designers of the Quaker Oats Company.

By 1893, the Quaker symbol had undergone subtle changes. Printing of the trademark in color on boxes inspired a redesign. The gaunt and austere Quaker gave way to a genial, fat bellied one, more ostentatious than any Friend would permit – with a red vest under the blue tailored coat, and golden buckles on his patent leather shoes. In this role he was a familiar resident of the American scene for many years. So too was the Quaker package, an acknowledged improvement over the unsanitary barrel which began to vanish from stores, and in its place, neat rows of 2-lb. packages of oats appeared on the shelves.

Seven decades later, Quaker Oats Company boasts over half a billion dollars worth of annual sales of more than 200 products, advertised in 16 languages, in 40 different countries. Oats are still one of their most nutritious products. Hopefully the company, one of the pillars in American food products, will stress nutrition values in all its products, and specifically childrens' cereals. Quaker Oats Company, we are sure, will want to continue its tradition of producing the best nourishment in all of its food products.

Arthur F. Marquette. *Brands, Trademarks and Good Will. The Story of the Quaker Oats Company.* New York: McGraw-Hill, 1967.

cereals became America's sensational business success story – plus a bonanza for dentists in filling and extracting rotten teeth caused by these sugared foods.

The testimony before the Senate Consumer Subcommittee on nutritional content and advertising for dry breakfast cereals* shows that children under 13 years who are moderate TV viewers spend over 1,000 hours a year in front of TV sets – more time than they spend with their teachers at school. They see over 5,000 TV advertisments per year for edible products alone – an average of over 100 minutes of TV commercials a week, mainly on foods and confections.

Average American children see over 80,000 TV food ads by the time they are 16 years old. Further, the foods advertised to them are not meats, fruits, vegetables, and dairy products – good foods that we all respect. They are mainly cereals and candies touted for their sweetness, glitter, and fun.

The studies show that it is only a short jump from the children's TV programs to mamma buying the puny breakfast cereals in the supermarket. Dr. Scott of Harvard University, in a study of these relationships, found that children score nearly 90% in pursuading their mothers to buy the advertised cereals. His chart is as follows:

Per cent of mothers usually yielding to child's purchase influence attempts

Breakfast cereals	88%
Snack foods	52%
Candy	40%
Soft drinks	38%

Dr. Ward Scott. *Television Advertising and Intra-family Influence.* Senate Consumer Subcommittee Hearings (Unpublished paper). March 2, 1972.

The plight of supermarket managers

Supermarket managers are virtually helpless in the face of these market forces. Breakfast cereal companies are paying over $50 million a year for TV advertising to push these mediocre breakfast foods.

The supermarket managers have no practical alternative but to display and sell them – or quit their jobs.

* Testimony by Council on Children, Media and Advertising. March 2, 1972.

And it is poor business. The 50 or 60 kinds of dry cereals occupy from 100 to 300 square feet of valuable supermarket space. They are low-profit items at the retail level, often yielding less than 10% in gross profit margin and sometimes as low as 3% on heavily advertised products such as Kaboom and Captain Crunch. Some supermarkets actually lose money on their dry breakfast cereal lines.

The true values of breakfast cereals

The big profits in breakfast cereals are made by the national food companies and their advertising agencies, not by the food retailers. If consumers would insist on cleaning up America's breakfast food mess and getting sensible stocks of nutritious merchandise on the supermarket shelves, the store managers would probably applaud such action and support it.

In six hours that same Saturday, CBS ran 126 commercials of which 87% were once again for edible products. And if a child had gotten up at 8:00 that morning and turned on CBS, he would have seen no commercials for anything except food and vitamins until after 9:00. In other words, by the time his folks crawled out of bed to feed him breakfast, he would have already been subjected to 27 ardent salesmen trying to tempt him to eat their products.

Which products? We have now analyzed the distribution of the 319 network food commercials which ran on the 29 hours of children's TV during the week we sampled. The chart I have here shows the distribution of ads into product categories.

Breakfast cereals	38½ %
Cookies, candy, gum, popcorn and other snacks	17 %
Vitamins	15 %
Beverages and beverage mixes	8 %
Frozen waffles and pop-tarts	7½ %
Canned pasta	5 %
Canned desserts, frozen dinners, drive-ins, peanut butter, oranges	9 %
Total	100 %

Joan Gussow, Nutritionist, Testimony before Senate Subcommittee on theConsumer. March 2, 1972.

WHOLE FOODS FOR YOU

Over the years that I had gone to the supermarket, I had watched it turn from a food store into an amusement park. I watched juice drinks, juice cocktails and dry powdered breakfast mixes crowd out fruit juices on the grocery shelf. I watched the frozen food cabinets expand to fill aisle after aisle offering the casual shopper everything from a frozen instant omelett for breakfast to a frozen Hero sandwich for lunch and frozen chow mein for dinner.

I saw the shelves fill up with an overwhelming array of cookies, crackers, breakfast cereals, soft drinks – and snacks and snacks and snacks. Everything from Bugles to Funions, from Onyums to Screaming Yellow Zonkers – and fake bacon made out of bargain basement soybeans to sell at Fifth Avenue prices.

All I knew at the time was that the things I wanted to buy were occupying a smaller and smaller proportion of stores that were growing larger and larger.

During these years I watched children I knew growing up on snacks – munching from bags of chips, or crackles or pops or chews, dipping into boxes of breakfast cereals made in nursery school colors and intensely sweet and artificial flavors. These same children were always too full for lunch or dinner or whatever meal it was they were supposed to eat. I watched mothers, affluent middle-class mothers, take their pre-schoolers to the park with a bag of miniature donuts and a bottle of juice drink for the child's lunch.

Joan Gussow. Op. cit.

The food values of dry cereals

Typical dry cereals are heavily processed grains, from which nearly all nutrients have been removed except for starch and protein. They then act as carriers for small amounts of synthetic vitamins and minerals, added during the manufacturing processes. They are, generally speaking, mediocre protein foods with low **protein efficiency ratios** (PERS).

A protein efficiency ratio (PER) is a comparison of protein in a particular food with that of an excellent protein food, such as milk or eggs. Whole milk, for example, has a PER rating of 2.5. Whole wheat by comparison has a protein value of 1.19, and the PER rating of whole oats is 1.98. The PER rating of Wheaties, in dismal contrast, is only .22. Country Corn Flakes and Stax have zero (0) protein values.

The true values of breakfast cereals

The principal additive to breakfast cereals is sugar. An analysis of sugared cereals by Robert B. Choate, Chairman of the Council on Children, Media and Merchandising (1346 Connecticut Avenue, N.W., Washington, D.C. 20036), showed the following amounts of sugar in several popular cereals:

Product	Cereal grains	Sugar
Kellogg Cocoa Krispies	45–50%	40–45%*
Kellogg Sugar Frosted Flakes	55–60%	30–35%*
Kellogg Special K	60–70%	30–35%*
General Mills Trix	50–60%	30–35%*
General Mills Frosty O's	40–45%	40–45%*
General Mills Count Chocula	35–40%	over 40%*
Quaker Oats Captain Crunch	49%	41%
Quaker Oats Quangaroos	43%	43%
Quaker Oats King Vitaman	33%	47%
General Foods Fruity Pebbles	48%	47%
General Foods Cocoa Pebbles	46%	46%
General Foods Alpha Bits	44%	42%
General Foods Super Sugar Crisp	42%	43%

* Calculated values. Figures not provided by the companies.

The current retail prices of these breakfast cereals are about 70¢ a pound. The retail price of sugar is about 13¢ a pound. The advertising investments by major food companies have the net result of conning customers into paying 700¢ extra for the sugar in their cereal products.

Fortification of breakfast cereals

The nutrients added to breakfast cereals by the manufacturers may include thiamin (vitamin B_1), riboflavin (vitamin B_2), niacin (a B vitamin), iron, and lysine (an amino acid protein unit), and even vitamins A, D, and C. When such nutrients are added, the amounts must be shown on the label – on the cereal boxes.

The new Food and Drug Administration labeling regulations provide that nutritional claims for fortified foods may be made only when the food contains the added nutrients in a significant quantity per regular serving. The minimum required level in such a serving must be at least 10% of the U.S. recommended daily allowance (RDA) if a value is claimed for the nutrient in the food.

For example, if a cereal manufacturer wishes to claim a thiamin (vitamin B_1) value in the product, the amount per breakfast serving must be at least .15 milligrams, since the recommended daily allowance for thiamin is 1.5 (and 1/10 of 1.5 equals .15).

In the case of iron, the manufacturer can claim a nutritional value if a breakfast serving contains at least 1.8 milligrams of iron, this being 1/10 of the official RDA of 18 milligrams.

It is hoped that these new labeling regulations will stimulate more honesty in advertising, labeling, and selling breakfast cereals.

Even when fortified, the major brands of dry breakfast cereals are generally poor, devitalized foods offering mainly starch and sugar at high prices. The vitamins and minerals in them, when present, are usually added synthetically, without regard to other nutritive factors, and have doubtful overall food values. The protein score is usually low when compared with protein in such foods as eggs, meat, and milk.

Good breakfast cereals

Life is being turned around in America, so we are seeking positive values to fill big voids shown in the 1940 – 1970 styles of living. Tired of gimmicks, gyps, and con games, millions of people are anxious to cut down the overhead costs in both time and money needed to live successfully for a day, a month, a year, and a lifetime.

They are even tired of complaining about "the system" and about phony breakfast cereals. They say, "Forget it. Give us something good, honest, and reasonably cheap."

Granola and whole cereals are part of the answer. We are back again to the unique values of seeds, grains, and nuts.

§ §

Food labeling for fortified breakfast cereals and other foods

The new Food and Drug Administration regulations, published March 14, 1973, state under Title 1.17 Food: Nutrition Labeling:

The following U.S. Recommended Daily Allowances (U.S. RDA) and nomenclature are established for these vitamins and minerals, essential in human nutrition:

Vitamin A, 5,000 International Units.	Vitamin B_6, 2.0 milligrams.
Vitamin C, 60 milligrams.	Folic acid, 0.4 milligram.
Thiamine, 1.5 milligrams.	Vitamin B_{12}, 6 micrograms.
Riboflavin, 1.7 milligrams.	Phosphorus, 1.0 gram.
Niacin, 20 milligrams.	Iodine, 150 micrograms.
Calcium, 1.0 gram.	Magnesium, 400 milligrams.
Iron, 18 milligrams.	Zinc, 15 milligrams.
Vitamin D, 400 International Units.	Copper, 2 milligrams.
Vitamin E, 30 International Units.	Biotin, 0.3 milligrams.

Pantothenic acid, 10 milligrams.

These nutrients and levels have been derived by the Food and Drug Administration from the "Recommended Dietary Allowances," published by the Food and Nutrition Board, National Academy of Sciences-National Research Council, and are subject to amendment from time to time as more information on human nutrition becomes available.

(v) No claim may be made that a food is a significant source of a nutrient unless that nutrient is present in the food at a level equal to or in excess of 10 percent of the U.S. RDA in a serving (portion). No claim may be made that a food is nutritionally superior to another food unless it contains at least 10 percent more of the U.S. RDA of the claimed nutrient per serving (portion).

(d) Products with separately packaged ingredients or to which other ingredients are added by the user may be labeled as follows:

Federal Register. U.S. Government
Printing Office. March 14, 1973, p. 6960.

Granola

Granola is a trade name for a class of foods made from whole seeds, grains, nuts, and even fruits, such as raisins. It is lightly processed, cooked moderately if at all, and can be eaten either dry or with milk as a breakfast cereal. The following is a high-quality granola recipe:

- 7 cups of old-fashioned oatmeal
- 1 cup of shredded coconut
- ¾ cup raw, shelled sunflower seeds
- ½ cup raw sesame seeds
- ½ cup sliced almonds
- 1 cup raw cashew nuts
- ½ cup honey
- ¼ cup good food oil
- 1 cup wheat germ
- 1 cup raisins

Mix the oatmeal, coconut, sunflower seeds, sesame seeds, almonds and cashews together. Pre-mix the honey and the cooking oil. Then mix these with the dry ingredients, above. Roast the raisins lightly, for 5 or 10 minutes in a 300 degree oven. Add them and the wheat germ, and mix the whole.

Spread about ¾ inch thick on cookie sheets and bake at 325 degrees for 10 or 15 minutes, or until the top is toasted a golden brown. Cool it, and tuck it away in cookie jars or where-ever you wish.

The cooking process is adequate to roast the raw seeds and cashew nuts.

Crunchy granola offered in food stores is usually less rich than this recipe since manufacturers aim for competitive prices on their products. They will put in more oatmeal and less of the higher-cost ingredients if needed to achieve a moderate price. The usual price of granola is about 75¢ a pound.

A Swiss product called Familia, a good quality granola, is often sold in U.S. food markets for about $1.30 a pound ($1.05 per 13-oz. package).

A nutrient analysis of granola shows that it is superior to any of the leading fortified dry cereals on the market.

A comparison of a typical granola product with the average of three leading brands of fortified cereals is as follows:

	Calories	Protein Per Cent	Riboflavin Mgs./Oz.	Niacin Mgs./Oz.	Iron Mgs./Oz.
Granola	350	11.9	1.8	1.2	3.9
Fortified Dry Cereals	110	4.9	.4	3.3	2.4

The true values of breakfast cereals

This granola food was priced at 70¢ a pound – a bit lower than the average prices of the fortified dry cereals.

We have found, in our own experience, that many children will accept granola if it is offered frequently and if the children are told of its advantages as a good food for them.

Granula

Granola originated many years ago under the name of "granula."

It was invented by Dr. Caleb Jackson, a Grahamite, abolitionist, water-cure doctor, lecturer, and founder of the health resort at Danville, New York. He attained fame in about 1850 for promotion of bloomers as the "American Costume" for women.

Dr. Jackson made *granula* with graham flour and water in a spartan recipe that contained little else.

Dr. J. H. Kellogg, soon after he organized the Battle Creek Sanitarium in 1877, prepared the first Battle Creek health foods, the Kellogg cereals. He called one of the first of these "granula" inspired by Jackson's invention. Upon being sued by Jackson, Kellogg changed the name of his product to "granola." The Kellogg granola was prepared from a mixture of wheat, corn and oat meals, mixed with water and seasoning, and baked a long time at a low oven temperature.

Dr. Kellogg liked the "grano" sound so well that he named his next breakfast cereal "granose." Made of cooked and rolled wheat flakes, it is one of the ancestors of "Wheaties."

Gerald Carson. From *Cornflake Crusade*.
New York: Rinehart and Company, Inc., 1957.

Try eating cereal boxes

There is a rather humorous and yet very telling experiment that Dr. William Caster, Professor of Nutrition, University of Georgia, did in the fall of 1970.

He recognized the milk-must-be-added arguments of the cereal company nutritionists who appeared here in August of 1970, and he asked the students to grind up the cardboard front of some of the cereal boxes, and to add sugar, milk, and raisins, and feed the mixture to a group of rats.

He said, "We then added one part of the box, one part sugar, one part of dry skim milk, and one part raisins by weight to a Waring blender and shredded these components together. This box diet was fed to another group of animals and the results would place this diet low in group B [that I have just described], but distinctly above group C."

In other words, he said that the cardboard box with milk and raisins and sugar would allow some growth, but was definitely superior to those cereals that fell in the category of little or no growth even when supplemented with a complete vitamin and mineral mixture. "When cardboard, which is normally thrown away, provides more nourishment than processed grains at 60 or 80 cents a pound, I think it is time to take a second look at who shapes this nation's nutrition."

Dr. Caster's nutritional evaluations of major dry cereal products, using laboratory rats as the indicators, were as follows:

Sunflower and pumpkin seeds

The turn toward granola in recent years is an advertisement for two of its possible ingredients: sunflower and pumpkin seeds. They revive our knowledge of the values of edible seeds as excellent human foods.

Again, it is the genius of seed foods that they contain the natural assortments of many nutrients to feed living things: plants, birds, animals, and people. Among the most valuable of these nutrients, so difficult to obtain in conventional American

Group A. Promotes excellent tissue growth:

Fortified Oat Flakes (Post) | Life (Quaker)

Group B. Allow some growth (less than half of the A group):

Concentrate (Kellogg)	Shredded Wheat (Nabisco)
Peanut Butter Crunch (Quaker)	Special K (Kellogg)

Group C. Little or no growth even when supplemented with a complete vitamin and mineral mixture:

Bran and Prune Flakes (General Foods)	Kaboom (General Mills)
Cherrios (General Mills)	Lucky Charms (General Mills)
Crispy Critters (General Foods)	Raisin Bran (Post)
Fruit Loops (Kellogg)	Rice Chex (Ralston)
Honey Comb (General Foods)	Total (General Mills)
Jets (General Mills)	Wheaties (General Mills)

Group D. Will not support life even when supplemented with a complete vitamin mixture and mineral mixture:

Apple Jacks (Kellogg)	Quisp (Quaker)
Clackers (General Mills)	Rice Crispies (Kellogg)
Corn Chex (Ralston)	Rice Honeys (Nabisco)
Corn Flakes (Kellogg)	Sugar Smacks (Kellogg)
Crunch Berries (Quaker)	Sugar Pops (Kellogg)
40% Bran Flakes (Kellogg)	Team (Nabisco)
Frosted Flakes (Kellogg)	Toasties (Post)
King Vitaman (Quaker)	Trix (General Mills)
Product 19 (Kellogg)	Wheat Chex (Ralston)
Puffed Wheat (Quaker)	Wheat Honeys (Nabisco)

Robert B. Choate, Chairman, Council on Children, Media And Merchandising. Testimony before Senate Subcommittee on the Consumer. March 2, 1972

diets, are the oil-soluble vitamins: A, D, E, and K.

Dr. Hal T. Slover of the Human Nutrition Research Division, USDA, found sunflower seeds to be quite high in vitamin E. These seeds had about four times as much vitamin E, for example, as corn and soybean seeds. The high vitamin E score for this seed food is, we believe, only an index to the underresearched values in such seeds as sunflower, pumpkin, sesame, and safflower.

Nutrients in sunflower, pumpkin and wheat seeds,

nutrients per pound

	Hulled sunflower seeds	Hulled pumpkin seeds	Red winter whole wheat
Calories	2,540	2,508	1,479
Protein, grams	109	131	46
Fat, grams	215	212	9
Carbohydrate, grams	90	68	327
Calcium, milligrams	544	231	191
Phosphorus, milligrams	3,797	5,189	1,814
Iron, milligrams	32	16	16
Potassium, milligrams	4,173	—	1,706
Vitamin A, I.U.	230	320	—
Thiamin (B_1), milligrams	8.9	1.11	1.95
Riboflavin (B_2), milligrams	1.05	.86	.50
Niacin, milligrams	24.7	10.8	16.3

Composition of Foods. USDA Handbook No. 8. 1963.

Fairly good packaged dry cereals

Mother's protests against the ridiculous sugar-frosted dry cereals and an increasing interest in better supermarket foods have stimulated food companies to make and offer some fairly good, new breakfast cereal products. These, plus the old standbys, such as Grape Nuts, Corn Flakes, Bran Flakes, Shredded Wheat, and Rice Crispies, make up an intermediate breakfast food group – some fairly good, nutritionally, and some just so-so.

The listing of ingredients on the labels is the guide for assessing these products. Grape Nuts, for example, shows up quite well, being made of:

Wheat, malted barley, salt, yeast, vitamin C, Niacin, Iron, Vitamin A, Vitamin B_6, vitamin B_2, vitamin B_1, vitamin D and vitamin B_{12}.

This is a straightforward, honest food, made of materials that are known to be good for people – certainly not harmful. The price, at 56¢ for 18 ounces, results in a cost of 3.2¢ an ounce.

In contrast, a highly promoted dry cereal called Total sells for 47¢ per 8 ounces, costing about 6¢ an ounce – nearly twice as much per ounce as Grape Nuts. It has the following ingredients, and bear in mind that they are **always** listed by order of decreasing amounts:

The true values of breakfast cereals

Whole wheat, sugar, salt, malt syrup, sodium ascorbate, sodium phosphate, calcium phosphate, niacin, iron, gum acacia, artificial color, vitamin E acetate, vitamin A palmitate, riboflavin, pyrodoxine (vitamin B_6), thiamin, calcium pantothenate, vitamin D and vitamin B_{12}. Freshness preserved by BHT.

At least 25% of this abominable breakfast food is sugar – sold for 90¢ a pound. Grape Nuts, by comparison, is a gorgeous food at half the price.

Old-fashioned Shredded Wheat, Corn Flakes, and Rice Crispies come out fairly well in the ingredients test – although sugar is being added to many of these older-name products. Shredded Wheat is still a straight cereal, free of added sugar.

The good newcomers

Health food awareness in America has brought some good newcomers to the dry cereal shelves. Granola and familia are the new models. In addition, these are of interest:

- **Quaker 100% Natural Cereal.** Made of brown sugar, whole wheat, raisins, dates, almonds, coconut, honey, oil, and dry milk, it is really a granola offered as a dry breakfast cereal or for snacking. Costs 75¢ for 18 oz. – about 4¢ an ounce.

- **Alpen,** an English product sold by Colgate-Palmolive, contains whole wheat, oats, dry milk, brown sugar, raisins, hazelnuts, almonds, malt, and salt. Again, a good quality granola-type product. Costs 68¢ for 12 ounces – about 5½¢ an ounce.

- **Heartland,** by Pet, Inc., is made of rolled oats, brown sugar, defatted wheat germ, oil, corn syrup, raisins, vanilla, sea salt and, lecithin. Costs 69¢ for 16 ounces – 4¼¢ an ounce.

- **Swiss Familia** is made of oats, apple flakes, whole wheat, rye, raisins, sugar, honey, almonds, and wheat germ concentrate. It is 89¢ per 12 ounces – about 7½¢ an ounce.

WHOLE FOODS FOR YOU

These fairly good breakfast cereals offer mothers a chance to help their children "kick the habit" of the bad kinds, so highly promoted with TV advertising, that rot their teeth and help to dwarf their bodies.

Cooked breakfast cereals – the old stand-bys

The little shelf next to the big dry cereal department in the food stores is the haven of the old stand-bys – the cereals to cook at home. It offers Rolled Oats, Cream of Wheat, grits, farina, Wheatena, and other do-it-yourself breakfast foods. This food line is growing in many stores, as customers become more informed about their foods.

The cooked cereals nearly always provide more nutrition, ounce for ounce and pound for pound, than the heavily advertised dry cereals. And they are much cheaper. For example, the enriched, sugared corn flakes, shown in the accompanying analysis of key food values, have less than one-third of the nutrition provided by oatmeal at over double the price.

Key values in oatmeal, farina and cornflakes

(per pound of food)

	Oatmeal	Farina	Corn Flakes Enriched	Corn Flakes Enriched and Sugar-covered
Calories	1,769	1,683	1,751	1,751
Protein, grams	64	52	36	20
Fat, grams	34	4	2	1
Carbohydrates, grams	309	349	387	414
Calcium, milligrams	240	113	77	54
Phosphorus, milligrams	1,837	845	204	109
Iron, milligrams	20	13	6	4
Potassium, milligrams	1,597	316	544	—
Thiamin (B_1), milligrams	2.7	2.0	1.9	1.9
Riboflavin (B_2)	.64	1.2	.36	.16
Approximate overall rating, if oatmeal is assigned a value of 100%.	100%	60%	40%	30%
Price per pound (1973, Washington, D.C.).	.32	.36	.37	.66

Nutrient values from *Composition Of Foods.* USDA Handbook No. 8, 1963

Examples of good hot cereals

Cooked whole grain cereals are the bargains in breakfast foods. The finest ones, available in nearly all food markets, are oatmeal and ready-to-cook whole wheat, in such products as Quaker Oats, Wheatena, and Ralston. These breakfasts cost about 5¢ per serving and are very nutritious. The following are examples of some of the good guys in cooked cereals:

Product	Description
Oatmeal or rolled oats (instant or regular)	Made of whole oat grains, high in protein, vitamin B complex, and food minerals. Has good iron content.
Wheatena	Made of whole wheat. Is equal to oatmeal in nutrients.
Ralston	Made of whole wheat with wheat germ added. Equal to Wheatena and oatmeal.
Cream of Wheat	This is a farina-type cereal, made of processed wheat. Not quite as high in nutrients as the whole grain products.
Farina	Same as Cream of Wheat.
Maltex	A blend of toasted wheat and barley flakes. Has good nutrient values.

All of these products, and others like them, are honest and economical breakfast foods. Most children will learn to like some of them, if given a good chance.

Logic, price, nutrition, honesty, and good sense favor selection of the whole grain breakfast foods. They cost half as much and are twice as good for you. We are aware, however, that food selection and eating are often illogical procedures in life. For many people, a bowl of frosted flakes is a delicious confection after a few days of eating good old oatmeal.

Our main point, perhaps, is that staple foods and candies are two entirely different products in any sound neighborhood operation and value system. When children are fed confections under food labels, confusion as well as tooth decay occurs, and family food costs that will be difficult to pay during the next era of high-cost American life.

§ §

A rogue's gallery of bad breakfast foods

(and many more are at large)

Learn to Read Breakfast Cereal Labels

These products are no worse than candies, cakes, pies, sodas, chewing gum, and sen-sen. They are desserts and confections. Don't get all riled up and try to kick them out of food markets – but put them in their proper places: in the candy and pastry departments. Do not offer them as staple breakfast foods for children or adults.

The following are examples of this whole group; there are many more. We hope they don't mind not being listed.

Remember, Federal law requires that the ingredients be listed in order of decreasing predominance in the product.

Kaboom contains sugar, oat flour, degermed yellow corn meal, corn syrup, wheat and corn starch, dextrose, salt, gelatin, coconut and peanut oils, sodium ascorbate, calcium carbonate, sodium phosphate, monoglycerides, artificial colors, niacin, iron, gum acacia, vitamin A palmitate, pyridoxine (vitamin B_6), riboflavin, thiamine, vitamin D, and vitamin B_{12}. Freshness preserved by BHT. Price 49¢ for 9 ounces – 5½¢ an ounce. Equals about 90¢ a pound for Kaboom.

Sugar Smacks contains sugar, wheat, corn syrup, hydrogenated vegetable oil, honey, salt, caramel color, sodium acetate, and lecithin with vitamins A and D in vegetable oil, sodium ascorbate, niacinamide, thiamine (B_1), riboflavin (B_2), pyridoxine (B_6), vitamin B_{12}, and iron phosphate added. BHA and BHT added to preserve product freshness. Price 41¢ for 10 oz. – 4¢ an ounce. Equals about 64¢ a pound for Sugar Smacks.

§ §

Lucky Charms contains oat flour, sugar and dextrose, corn syrup, wheat and corn starch, salt, gelatin, coconut and peanut oils, calcium carbonate, sodium phosphate, sodium ascorbate, artificial flavors, niacin, iron, gum acacia, vitamin A palmitate, pyridoxine (vitamin B_6), riboflavin, thiamine, vitamin D, and vitamin B_{12}. Freshness preserved with BHT. Price 47¢ for 9 ounces – a little more than 5¢ an ounce. Equals about 83¢ a pound.

Froot Loops contains sugar, corn, wheat and oat flour, hydrogenated vegetable oil, salt, certified colors and natural fruit flavoring with sodium ascorbate, vitamins A and D in vegetable oil, niacinamide, thiamine (B_1), riboflavin (B_2), pyridoxine (B_6), vitamin B_{12}, and iron phosphate added. BHA added to preserve product freshness. Price 57¢ for 11 oz. – about 5¢ an ounce. Equals about 82¢ a pound.

Boo Berry contains sugar, oat flour, degermed yellow corn meal, wheat and corn starch, dextrose, salt, corn syrup, coconut and peanut oils, gelatin, calcium carbonate, monoglycerides, sodium phosphate, sodium ascorbate, artificial flavors, artificial colors, niacin, iron, gum acacia, citric acid, vitamin A palmitate, pyridoxine (vitamin B_6), riboflavin, thiamine, vitamin D, and vitamin B_{12}. BHT added to preserve freshness. Price 47¢ for 8 oz. – a little less than 6¢ an ounce. Equals about 96¢ a pound. This cereal gets special mention because the label is deceptive: It indicates that the product contains blueberries – or at least some fraction of that fruit, and also bits of marshmallows; but neither of these materials – evidently – is in the product.

GUIDES AND SUGGESTIONS

Breakfast cereals

The realities of present-day life should be recognized: Commuters may not wish to rise 30 minutes early to have a cooked breakfast. Children will not suddenly cease watching Kid Power, Bugs Bunny, Pufn'stuf, Yogi's Gang, Deputy Dawg, Underdog, and Mr. Magoo on Saturday mornings. Big food companies will not suddenly get religion and promote low-profit good foods rather than high-profit nothing foods.

Meantime, we offer the following guides and suggestions:

1. Bring whole seeds, cereals, and grains into your personal and family diets, steadily and persistently, until these foods are in your life style and in the family eating pattern.

2. Put the heavily processed and sugared, boxed, dry cereals in their proper place – desserts, confections, and occasional foods to break the monotony of everyday eating.

3. Be patient with children and stubborn adults. Explain why the whole seeds and grains are needed in breakfasts, since it is so hard to get enough of their nutrients in other meals.

4. Sit with your children (if you have any) and watch several Saturday morning TV programs. Then send your sincere message, if you have one, to the food companies that advertise sugared and other poor breakfast cereals. Ask them to provide equal time for promotion of good foods and nutrition on children's TV programs.

5. Select from the new, fairly good quality dry breakfast cereals (such as those listed under The Good Newcomers) in helping your family to have variety in their breakfasts – and to shift away from the sugared dry cereals.

6. Eat cooked breakfast cereals at least once a week, and teach the children (if any) to eat them. Oatmeal, farina, Cream of Wheat, and Ralston are good examples to start with – and you will eventually find several more.

7. Select and eat hulled sunflower and pumpkin seeds, granola, and other seed foods. If your food store does not stock these products, ask the manager to do so, and explain why.

8. Seeds and granola are good snack foods as well as breakfast items. Have a bowl of them on your desk or at your work place for impulsive snacking. Or, eat some on the bus or train on the way to work, to finish your breakfast.

9. Rise above, go around, and under sugared and empty breakfast cereals. Don't fight them too hard; it wastes energy. They, too, will pass.

FOODGRAM No. 6

Seed foods for breakfast

Are You Looking for Ways to Break the Bad Breakfast Habit?

Then learn to eat granola, familia, and other seed foods, along with fruit juice for breakfast. These foods combine whole clusters of hard-to-get nutrients and feature the vitality factors: protein, oil, vitamins, and food minerals.

A good granola recipe is given on page ooo. Familia is a variation of granola, especially suited for breakfasts. Here is an attractive familia recipe:

Instant Familia

3 cups rolled oats
2 cups rolled wheat or other cereal
1 ½ cups raw wheat germ
3 cups powdered milk
1 cup chopped peanuts
½ cup chopped cashew or other nuts
1 cup sunflower seeds, hulled raw
1 cup pumpkin seeds, hulled raw
1 cup raisins (amount to suit taste)
1 cup dried chopped apricots, peaches, prunes, or other fruit
1 cup shredded coconut

Mix all ingredients together and store in refrigerator.

One advantage of this familia recipe is that you can add warm or hot water when the familia is served, and make a milk and cereal breakfast. This activates the powdered milk in the familia. Or eat the familia dry, as in eating granola.

SEEDS AND ORANGE JUICE

Seeds and orange juice make a good breakfast variation for busy people. Sunflower and pumpkin seeds are suitable for this purpose. Choose the hulled, raw kinds that are available in many food stores.

Simply pour the seeds into a convenient bowl and eat them by hand while drinking the orange juice and reading the morning paper – or being pleasant. Those with an addiction for work can have such a breakfast at their shop or office. Just munch the seeds and drink your juice.

One-third of a cup of these seeds (about 2 ounces) is a suitable portion for a morning meal. Reaching for them tends to be compulsive, and eating this amount takes about 15 minutes of pleasant chewing – reviving this lost art in American eating.

The seeds and juice provide about 400 calories – 300 in the seeds and 100 in the juice.

After 10 days of this kind of a breakfast, look out! Old women are beautiful, young ones are heavenly, and men of all ages bump into each other while looking back over their shoulders at passers-by.

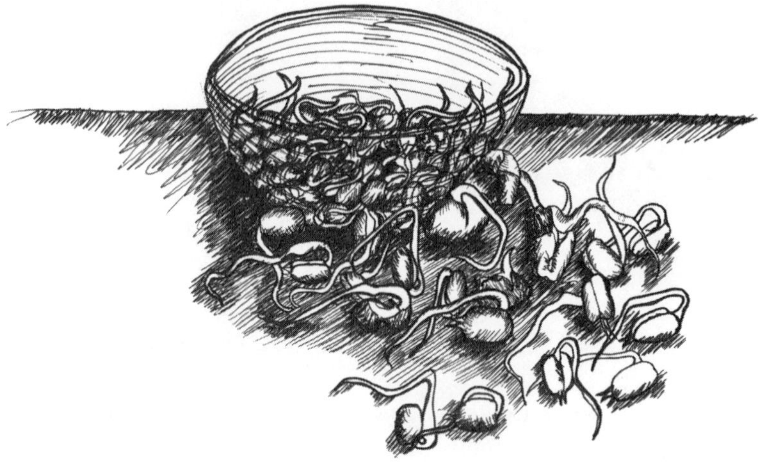

Seeds are akin to eggs in containing whole nutrition for life – everything needed by a new life unit until it is able to start gathering foods for itself. Chinese people learned many centuries ago that seed eggs are as useful as bird eggs in nourishing people. If the seeds are sprouted, they become live whole foods. The techniques for growing seed sprouts and eating them are given in this chapter.

Catharyn Elwood, America's beloved nutritionist and seed sprout expert, entered the nutrition field as a lay person in 1928, seeking to prevent dental carries and weak jawbones in children. She obtained nutrition education and an M.S. degree at the University of Maryland in 1943. Catharyn Elwood's best seller, *Feel Like a Million,* has sold over 750,000 copies. Students who pay homage to her live all over the United States. She is noted for being a gentle rebel in nutrition and foods.

7

Sprouts -

Live Whole Foods

Wouldn't you like something new, something delicious to eat? Some fresh, organic food chock-full of vitamins and life-giving enzymes for every meal? And without going shopping? Something succulent and crisp that has no waste, takes little or no time to prepare, that can be ready to eat in 3 to 5 days, grows any place and at any season of the year? A full-flavored food which rivals meat in protein and orange juice in vitamin C?

Or perhaps the best news of all if your food budget is shrinking is that sprouts, the highly nutritious food-for-life we are talking about, costs just pennies a day.

If there is such a thing as a miracle food on earth, most certainly it is sprouts, for all life depends on seeds and their successful growing for existence. Yes, plants, animals, and man, too.

Fortunate are we that this ancient art of sprouting seeds-for-food has been revived and that it is fast becoming the popular "in thing" for those who know and care about better foods for better health.

Quality seeds that still have their life, their "grow power," are vigorous sprouters. That makes it possible for everyone to have a flourishing, good-eating, indoor garden minus the five W's (weeding, watering, waiting, worrying, and work). All we need to do is provide the right environment of moisture, temperature, and ventilation.

Seeds thrive and grow everywhere if given half a chance. In snowbound villages, swamps, ghettos, mansions; in attics, cellars, bomb shelters, caves, or dugouts. They keep on doing their "divine thing" – just growing faithfully day after day, year after year.

"Sprouties for every meal" is our motto, and you can have them even if you are on the go. I know, for every once in a while traveling students or friends, who also have been bitten by this sprout thing, ring my bell to show me how they keep their sprout crop flourishing while "on the road." If hiking or biking, bags or cartons of these delicious nuggets of nutrition continue to grow, safely tucked in a backpack. Bus, train, or airplane trips offer no problems either; and by car, it is as easy as tucking your sprout-growing containers under your sink or on your windowsill at home.

Lucky are we sprout enthusiasts, for we never worry about the weather, pesticides, weedicides, herbicides, poison sprays, harsh chemical fertilizers, or any of the other contaminants, pollutants, and questionable additives of our modern food-growing and processing technology.

Best seeds for sprouting

The favorite seeds for sprout food are naturally the most delicious ones to eat and the easiest to grow. Mung beans, lentils, alfalfa, wheat, peas, and corn are favorites. I suggest you start with them. But all seeds that are used for food and will sprout can be used, except, of course, those chemically treated for planting. Test many. You will soon find your favorites and use them often.

Rye, oats, barley, millet of the grains and lentils, peas and chickpeas (garbanzos), soybeans (see success tips), navy beans, lima beans, white-, black-, and spotted beans – in fact, all of the legumes (seeds that grow in pods) are suitable. They make fine sprouts. Sunflower, buckwheat, radish, cress, turnip, clovers, lettuce, parsley, onions, beets, kale, fenugreek, and others add a most interesting variety of flavors from snappy and tart to mild and sweet. It is more difficult to grow nuts, but peanuts and almonds soaked overnight begin to sprout and become soft enough for all ages to enjoy. Drop the soaked almonds into scalding hot water for just a few seconds to loosen the skins. Then slip them off easily before serving.

Sprouts – live whole foods

What about containers?

Among many containers used for sprouting that I've seen or successfully used are the following: bottles with strainer lids, sink strainers, colanders, coffee percolators, a steamarvel, unglazed flower pots and dishes, terry cloth towels or face cloths (rag doll method), sponges, a small chest of 3 drawers (about 6 by 14 inches with hardware cloth wire mesh in the bottom of the drawers). This popular little sprout chest needed face cloths to put the seeds to bed and cover. One tap washing flooded all three drawers and draining was easy. Pretty salad or fruit bowls can be used with wire mesh bent at the corners to hold it about an inch from the bottom of the bowl. Over this rack, a white terry or firm-textured cloth was laid, over which the seeds were evenly spread. The cloth was cut long enough so that other half could be folded back to cover the seeds. The ends of the cloth were allowed to dip well into the water in the bottom, keeping the cloth evenly dampened at all times. Also, metal cans or milk cartons with holes punched in the bottom can be used. (One friend uses a large can with a handle to hang on the tap, and has cut a door on the side near the top for servicing the crop.) Cloth bags or an old sock fastened or tied to the water tap or dish drainer. This old-sock idea catches the imagination of the children and gives them a good lesson in nutrition if their help can be enlisted. After all, they hang up socks for Santa to fill. Why not let Mother Nature's nourishment be the gift until Christmas?

Certainly, equipment and gadgets are no problem. Many new gadgets are on the market – some fancy and expensive. They may be obtained from health food stores or through mail order houses.

How to sprout

The simplest, easiest apparatus I have found is the wide-mouthed pint, quart, 2-quart, or gallon glass jar. Place 1 teaspoon to 1 tablespoon of seeds (depending on the kind) in the

Summary on how to sprout seeds

The following suggestions should enable you to sprout seeds with a minimum amount of effort.

1. Select good seeds in any supermarket, health food store, specialty or garden store. The seeds you may choose from include peas, beans, alfalfa, wheat, mung beans, and lentils.

2. Select any container such as a deep dish, jar, bottle, milk carton, crock, or flower bowl. A few tablespoons of seeds should be placed in the container and soaked in water for 8 to 15 hours.* This will initiate sprouting, although some seeds take longer. Also, most seeds should be kept in the dark, and, therefore, containers should be kept covered. Keep germinating seeds at normal room temperature.

3. The water should be poured off of the soaked seeds. Thereafter, the seeds should be washed and drained morning and evening, or several times each day. The important point is that the seeds must be kept moist but not too wet after the initial period of soaking.

4. Once the sprouts appear, they may be eaten; however, ½ inch of sprout from the seed generally produces a sweet, fresh-tasting food. Adjust time of eating to your own taste, and kind of seed.

5. Keep sprouts refrigerated in a covered dish until used. They may be eaten raw, cooked, or mixed with many other kinds of food.

* If you wish larger amounts of sprouts, put more seeds into the container.

pint-sized jar and proportionately larger amounts in larger jars. Fill jar ¼ to ½ full of lukewarm pure water. A netting nylon, very small mesh, is best for covering the top of the jar. A double net is needed for the tiny seeds. Fasten with an elastic band or string around the neck of the jar. Soak overnight or longer. Leaving the net on the jar, pour soaking water off in the morning. Drink or save the water (in which the seeds were soaked) for cooking. Place jar under the tap and refill. Then very gently, shake the jar in a rotary motion to separate seeds and tip the jar to allow the water to drain out. Placing on a dish drainer to allow complete drainage is the easiest method.

In the evening, repeat the rinsing of the seeds. Remember that the seeds must be kept moist – but not standing in water or they will rot. If allowed to get dry, the seeds will not sprout.

The sprouts will be ready to eat when you enjoy them the most. Wheat is best when the length of the sprout is no longer than ½ inch; lentils, peas, and soy beans when about 1 to 1½ inches; alfalfa, radish, red clover, and fenugreek when 1 to 2 inches; and mung beans, if grown to perfection, can get 2 to 3 inches, improving in flavor, nourishment, and crispness all the way.

Chill your tender young sprouts by rinsing in a pan of cold water. Most of the cellulose seed coatings will float off or sink to the bottom so the bulk of them can be discarded, although they no doubt offer good roughage for colon health too. Eat all sprouts while fresh or place them in closed jars or bags and refrigerate as any fresh vegetable.

Other covers, except cloth, may be used for jars or containers. Very fine, stainless steel wire mesh to fit the top and held on with Mason jar rim, cheesecloth, gauze, and so forth may be used also, or the top of a nylon stocking – in fact, anything that drains well will do.

Experiment a bit and you will find that sprouts grow faster and become longer in the dark. Put them in light or a sunlit spot when you wish green leaves to develop. This is important for alfalfa and clovers. Then chlorophyl, vitamin A, magnesium, iron, and other health values appear with the green leaves and make for sumptuous eating.

One word of warning to eat-every-kind-of-sprout enthusiasts – do not eat potato sprouts. They have a toxic element that is not healthful.

When and how to use sprouts

Use sprouts as soon as they are at their best. They are best served raw, but many prefer to cook them very lightly or blended for unusual dishes. They may be used for all salads, soups, chop suey and other Oriental dishes, casseroles, breakfast cereals, breads, waffles, rolls and other baked goods; egg or meat dishes; sandwich spreads, sprout milks, ice creams, snacks, and candy – in fact, every type of food is improved by adding sprouts.

Helpful suggestions on how to use sprouts

Bean Sprouts. Soybeans, limas, navy, pinto, or the whole world of other beans may be sprouted and used in your favorite recipes. The only thing to remember is that the sprouted bean is already softened and doesn't need overnight baking (baked beans, brown, for instance) to make a well-done dish. The longer you cook them and the higher the heat, the greater the loss of perishable vitamins and sensitive enzymes we hunger for everyday. So use your favorite recipes, enhanced by flavor from sprout food and goodness, but be wary of overcooking. The additional natural flavors will please everyone.

Alfalfa Sprouts. It is a pity to cook the crisp, tender sprouts of alfalfa and other growing vegetables. The alfalfa makes such a delectable lettuce substitute in sandwich filling – be sure and pile thick – or use as a bed for any salad, including avocado. Once while attending a luncheon meeting, I commented on the pale, winter iceberg lettuce. The lady next to me said: "We never buy lettuce in the winter. We depend on alfalfa sprouts completely for our greens in salads. They are pure, dependable every day of the year, and we think they are more delicious." She then went into quite a story about them, how, by themselves, they are wonderful with your favorite dressing.

Mung and Lentils. These and other sprouts can be used raw in salads, or dropped into your favorite soup just before serving. Rye sprouts taste like wild rice. They may be used in salads and for all types of sandwiches. They are added to every type of stew, casseroles, and even souffles.

Grain Sprouts. These sprouts, particularly wheat, rye, oats, barley, and rice are especially delicious. Bread, waffles, pancakes, in fact all baked goods, are improved with the addition of grain sprouts. The sprout may become the dough without the addition of any flour (see bread recipe). Nut-flavored sprouts may be added as one would add chopped nuts. The flavor is tremendously improved, the texture made more chewy, and you already know the improvement in nutrition.

The sprouting act – success tips

One most interesting thing about growing sprouts is that each variety of seed behaves differently. You have to know what to expect as they grow to help them along. Experience is your best teacher, so don't be discouraged if one time you do not get as luxurious sprouts as you want. Try to improve your care and undertaking of them. Here are some tips that should improve your technique.

1. Seed quality. If two or more failures occur, and you have been careful in providing proper care, return your seeds (if you can) and ask the store manager if he will please get you seeds that will sprout.

2. Environment. Check the environment of the seeds. Is the water pure? Some seeds are sensitive to chlorine and fluorine.

3. Temperature. What is the temperature? If the kitchen gets cold at night in the winter, many seeds thrive with the change of temperature, but others do not like the change and do much better when the temperature is maintained near 70°. If you have a pilot-lighted gas stove, the pot and pan area under it may be a better place to store your sensitive sprouts while growing. Or, if you have a warm corner near the furnace pipes, that may prevent chilling on cold nights. Put your sprout chest, bottles, or whatever near the warm place.

Some eager sprouters contrive a low-watt light bulb in a box for the sprout equipment. You will think up other methods that will work for you.

4. Moisture. What about the moisture? All sprouts must be kept damp, but well drained. You must tip the jars, if they are your chosen equipment, so the water drains out completely or the seeds will rot standing in the water. To prevent drying out between washings, you may find it necessary to place a wetted paper towel or small cloth over the top of them. Check your method of sprouting.

Some easy-molding and rotting beans need more frequent washings. Twice or three times a day is usually enough, but the protein-rich beans do better with four or more gentle washings to clean them.

5. Special tips for soybeans. In sprouting soybeans, the Chinese use a bleaching agent, such as highly diluted chlorox. We have a natural herbal wash, equisetrum (horsetail) herb that prevents mold even more effectively. Some health food stores and herb specialty shops carry it, and it will not harm tender growing sprouts. Made as a tea, it is also a healthful beverage. One teaspoon of equisetrum is added to 1 cup of boiling water. Steep for 15 minutes or longer. For washing soybean sprouts and preventing mold, it can be diluted at the rate of 1 teaspoon to 2 quarts of water. It may be used over and over as the only wash for soybeans during their growing period of 5 or 6 days.

Sprouts provide free vitamins

Sprouts double, triple, and quadruple, and sometimes increase vitamins hundreds of times over. For instance, 1 tablespoon of alfalfa seeds gives you a quart of excellent sprouts. But this generous increase in amount cannot compare with the bonanza of life-saving vitamins they supply at the same time. These versatile sprout vitamins seem to play hide-and-seek during growth. Researchers find them one day and then they disappear, only to reappear with a supercrop the third day. This could account for some of the confusion regarding reports on vitamins in sprouts. If a researcher tests on a low day, he reports "no vitamins." This happened to Dr. Pauline Berry Mack who used soybeans for a vitamin study. In 24 hours, there was no vitamin A, but after 72 hours, they had poured forth an abundance of this vitamin.

Sprouts and vitamin C

If you choose wheat or other grains – which are easy to sprout – you will be getting a whopping increase of 600% in vitamin C during the very early growing period. If you are eating soybeans, the beefsteak of China, vitamin C content has skyrocketed 550% in 72 hours. Oats are a bit slower, but vitamin C has increased from 11 to 43 milligrams in 5 days. Where else can you get a 300% increase in food values? Dried peas sprouted – another delicious favorite – offer you 69 milligrams of vitamin C in every 100 grams. This increases to 86 milligrams in 4 days. Here is a vitamin-growing timetable for peas and oats from England.

Sprouts – live whole foods

Do you remember your vitamin C lesson? Briefly, vitamin C works quickly in the body. If you are not getting enough vitamin C and are plagued with the common, subclinical scurvy symptoms of pink toothbrush, fatigue, easy bruising, slow healing, aching joints, annoying allergies, infections, sluggishness, and common colds, you may need more vitamin C. These problems should begin to fade away as you increase your vitamin C intake and begin to restore your resistance.

Vitamin C values of germinated seeds

	Milligrams in 100 grams
Oats, whole	11
after germination for 96 hours	20
after germination for 120 hours	42
Peas, dry	0
after germination for 24 hours	8
after germination for 48 hours	69
after germination for 96 hours	86

Reprinted from FEEL LIKE A MILLION by Catharyn Elwood by permission of The Devlin-Adair Company, Old Greenwich, Conn. Copyright 1956 by Catharyn Elwood.

Vitamin B complex in sprouts?

Each member of the vitamin B family seems to be competing for first sprouting honors. In sprouting oats, vitamin B_2 (riboflavin) wins first place by an upshot of 1,350% in 5 days. Vitamin B_1 (thiamine), well known for high energy, offers a 10% increase. Vitamin B_6 (pyridoxine), that has been stealing the vitamin show for 5 or 6 years and is known to be an essential part of many body enzyme systems, provides an increase of 500%. Folic acid does even better. It literally skyrockets 600% during sprouting. Niacin, now well known for mental health, provides 500% more, while biotin and pantothenic acid increase 200%. Nutritional science tells us that these simple little sprouts are health power packets. They have nourished thousands of people suffering from pellagra, beriberi, and scurvy back to health. (For details, see Chapter 35 in Feel Like a Million).

The health benefits of our vitamin B Complex may never be completely understood because life is so complex, but their high energy and contributions to disease resistance have made them famous. Never forget the vitamin B Complex feeding experiment at the University of Toronto. Animals were divided into two groups. One group got all the vitamin B Complex needed. The other group was short-changed. When disease-producing germs were injected into their B-deficient bodies, only 20% of them survived. Of those getting enough B Complex, 89% not only survived, but thrived.

Vitamin B complex increases in sprouting wheat and oats

	Per Cent Increase	
	Wheat	Oats
Thiamin (B_1)	20	10
Riboflavin (B_2)	450	1,350
Niacin	65	—
Pantothenic Acid	85	200
Pyridoxine	50	500
Biotin	100	50
Folic Acid	300	600

Feel Like a Million. *Op. cit.*

Sprouts provide highest quality protein

The supreme nourishment of a food is measured by its protein. "How long will it maintain life?" Perfect reproduction through successive generations is not possible if proteins are not complete in their building blocks, their amino acids composition. Regardless of what the test-tube researchers show or say about protein production from growing grains, sprouts have proven time and again that they maintain normal health through three successive generations. The late Dr. Francis Pottenger, Jr., of Monrovia, California, was the first to report this with controlled animal experiments.

It must be this same mysterious completeness that has restored fertility to sterile cattle. Reports come from many countries about "complete and successful rejuvenation," as well as from our own USDA at Beltsville, Maryland. Animals of both sexes that were less successful in reproduction became quite fertile and healthy. Fine, normal offspring resulted in all tests where the diet was controlled. Five pounds of sprouts, dry weight, and equal amounts of silage, were fed each animal for 60 days. Breeding then was successful in every animal.

Sprouts – live whole foods

In India, Dr. Rochanapuranda increased the total proteins contained in mung beans from 16.6% to 18.25% in 6 days, by sprouting. Dr. Johns, another researcher, found that 10% of the total protein was lysine. Lysine is the director of the whole protein amino acid symphony. The other amino acids (protein-building blocks) do not know what to do if lysine is not on the job. Vegetarian fare is often seriously deficient in lysine. This may be due to a predigesting of the proteins during sprouting.

Sprouts provide high nutritional values at very low cost

For those who do not digest starch easily during digestion, sprouts may be helpful. The starches are converted during sprouting to simple sugars, says Dr. Loa of China, thus making them an excellent quick-energy food. Sprouts are an easily digested food for everyone, including the weight-watchers.

The more sprouts you eat, the less your diet will cost. This means that the more bountiful your diet nutritionally, the less expensive it becomes. Sounds incredible, doesn't it? But just as sprouts grow the highest nutritional values, they shrink the costs of eating. Let's see if we can prove it.

Mung Beans. Just the other day, I saw some of these tiny green beans in a health food store in a barrel. You served yourself at 55¢ a pound. The usual packaged pound is about 75¢. (Do you remember when they were 20¢ to 25¢ a pound with few buyers?) Let's figure a pound at 75¢. One pound is about 2 cups or nearly 24 tablespoons. That means about 3¢ each. Two tablespoons, at 6¢, if cared for properly, will grow into a quart or more of sprouts. If you eat a full cupful, that is 1¼¢. Half a cup, an average serving, amounts to ¾ of a cent. Isn't this quite an inducement to serve them daily? Some of the best things in life, including sprouts, are "nearly free."

Alfalfa. One pound of these wee miracle seeds measures 2 cups or close to 24 tablespoons. The price has gone up recently from 75¢ to $1.60 which more than doubles the cost. Nevertheless, they are still at the bottom of the cost scale while standing high in nutrition. At 7¢ a tablespoon, that means 7¢ for a quart of sprouts. From this, one can get six to eight sizable salad nests, or near-Dagwood-sized fillings to replace lettuce of questionable quality and higher cost – little more than 1¢ a serving.

Wheat. All the grains are near the same price as wheat. The miller pays about 4¢ a pound in quantity. We pay near 50¢ in most stores. Twenty-four tablespoons averages a bit more than 2¢ each. It nearly doubles itself in soaking and when just right to eat as a delicious sprout cereal or in other food, it has increased 100% again. Two to 4 tablespoons makes a serving when combined with fruits, as in muesil. How much to serve depends on appetite and size of your stomach, besides what else is on the menu.

Catharyn Elwood's sprouts recipes

Sprout müsli This breakfast of sprouts, fruit, and nut müsli is very popular. I learned how to make it at the Bircher-Benner Sanitarium in Zurich, Switzerland, where they use "foods as medicine" and "cure the incurables." They demonstrated it in their famous kitchen and served our nutrition group the dish at teatime in the dining room.

The recipe. Wheat sprouts, ¼ to ½ cup. Other grains or mixture of grains can be used. (The sanitarium included some rolled oats that had been soaked overnight.)

One apple (organic preferred). Grate everything but the stem and pour over this the juice of one lemon. A little lime, grapefruit, or orange juice may be substituted, or the lemon can be omitted if not on hand. However, the juice prevents the apple from turning dark, as well as adding a good amount of vitamin C.

Add one tablespoon of soaked raisins. Other dried fruits may be used, or the dried fruits can be used in place of the apple, for a change. Bananas, fresh strawberries, fresh peaches, or any fresh fruit in season will give variety (in place of or with the apple) and make delightful combinations that will always whet your appetite!

Slivered almonds or pecans, filberts, or any other nut may also be used if desired. Sunflower or pumpkin seeds may be added or substituted for the nuts for interesting changes in flavors. The seeds and nuts are delicious if ground fine in a grinder, and as you know from the material on seeds and oils, these wonders of nature provide another whole food for you.

This dish is sweet enough to satisfy most tastes. If not sweet enough for you, add a spot of honey or pure maple syrup. If you prefer the mixture to be more moist, add milk, yogurt, or other cultured, or seed, or nut milks. Each will provide a different taste, and all are healthful.

Like all foods, this sprout dish should be chewed to a liquid that trickles down your throat. Every drop savored and enjoyed.

For additional variations of the sprout müsli, wheat germ or a small amount of your special granola may be added for flavor and interest. If you enjoy a hot, cooked, whole grain breakfast cereal, combine this cereal with some wheat or grain. You will like this combination too.

Remember this müsli dish can be served anytime of the day. The simple recipe of rolled oats soaked overnight with sprouts, apple, lemon, nuts, raisins, and milk is often served 3 times a day for certain beneficial effects at Birchner-Benner.

Sprout salads

You name your favorite salad; and I will tell you how to add sprouts to it, making it more enticing, tasty, and nourishing. For instance, any sprouted seed will blend well with the always-popular tossed salad. Favorite sprouts for this purpose include mung, alfalfa, lentil, fenugreek, or wheat. Fruit salads, regardless of the kind of dressing used, are made more appetite-whetting by adding delicate alfalfa sprouts about 1½ inches long, with their small, green caps ready to burst into leaf. Fenugreek, 2 inches long, is excellent. Fruits, such as apricots, peaches, and figs, soaked overnight and made plump again, are especially delicious with wheat sprouts. When about

½ inch long, they can easily take the place of nuts for flavor in this salad.

Crisp, fresh vegetable salads, whether mostly leafy greens or a combination of finely grated vegetables tossed together, are far more fun and tasty if mung bean sprouts are added. I grow mine 1½ to 2 inches long before the leaves appear. Lentils, fenugreek, alfalfa, or any ready-to-eat sprout may be tossed in at the last minute. Remember the rule of making tossed salads: After the leafy greens are washed, dried, and broken into pieces, they and the sprouts are oiled carefully and well. Then your snappy dressing doesn't wilt them on contact. They stay fresh and crisp if covered well in the refrigerator, even overnight.

A good sprout salad recipe is given in Food-Gram No. 4 on page 60.

Lentil sprout soup

Heat 1 quart soup stock and add:
2 cups sprouted lentils
1 medium onion, finely sliced or diced
1 medium-sized carrot, sliced or diced
1 or 2 stalks of celery, sliced
1 small potato, scrubbed well and grated
1 bay leaf
sea salt to please you
⅛ teaspoon (pinch) thyme
1 teaspoon lemon juice (added and stirred well just before serving)

Simmer over medium heat until lentils and vegetables are soft but not soggy. Remove bay leaf, add lemon juice, and serve.

And now – good luck! Many who really get into the sprouting thing have encouraging success from the very beginning . . . others call or write in despair of ever getting the knack of it. Don't give up, don't get discouraged. Try again and again . . . it might even be the wrong sign of the moon that makes it more difficult for you to succeed easily!

Indeed, you will be grateful and appreciate all your efforts when you can serve sprouts 3 times a day and for snacks between meals, too. Teach your club, church, or children at school how to proceed and succeed and maybe do as many have – go into a profitable, humanitarian type of business for yourself. Some have written that they have even kept the rather cute name of "Sprouties," and are now delivering them to all of the food stores in their town. Bless them! And you for your dedication and interest. You will thank me someday when you have kept at it long enough to feel ever-renewing energy and enjoy the saved money from food bills. It will help you to buy other good foods.

Sprouts – live whole foods

Quick and easy wheat sprout bread (flourless)

2 cups wheat berries (organic, if possible) soaked 24 hours. Change the soaking water every 8 hours. This will make about 4 cups of sprouted wheat.

Add:

1 package dried baker's yeast
2 – 4 tablespoons wheat germ flakes
1 teaspoon bone meal (or any calcium-rich product)
2 tablespoons lecithin granules
½ teaspoon powdered kelp
2 or 3 tablespoons honey

Let rise to double its bulk. With oiled hands, knead lightly and place in oiled bread pans. Let rise and bake as in any breadmaking.

If you want festive bread, add chopped dried fruits, raisins, figs, apricots, bananas, prunes, any or all. Also sesame, sunflower, pumpkin, or squash seeds may be added, plain or sprouted, any one or all. These will add flavor to any of your breads, and considerable nutrition. A little lemon juice can also be used to highlight flavors. Experiment with your foods. You may create a real favorite or winner.

Meats, poultry, and fish have been staple protein foods for Americans ever since we became a nation. Rising prices dictate that most people must curtail their purchases of these foods. One peril in such a change is that people will fail to get essential vitamins and minerals since meat foods are rich in these nutrients. However, an analysis shows that the vitamin and mineral values are mainly in the lean *meats, not in the* fat. *The featured USDA "Prime" and "Choice" meats are actually lower in essential nutrients than the cheaper "Good," "Standard," and "Commercial" grades. Selections of these lower grades are proper for better nourishment. Poultry and fish are also good providers of vitamins and minerals as well as protein-rich sources and should be selected.*

We analyze grades and kinds of meat in this chapter, and suggest ways to get protein, vitamins, and minerals in less expensive foods.

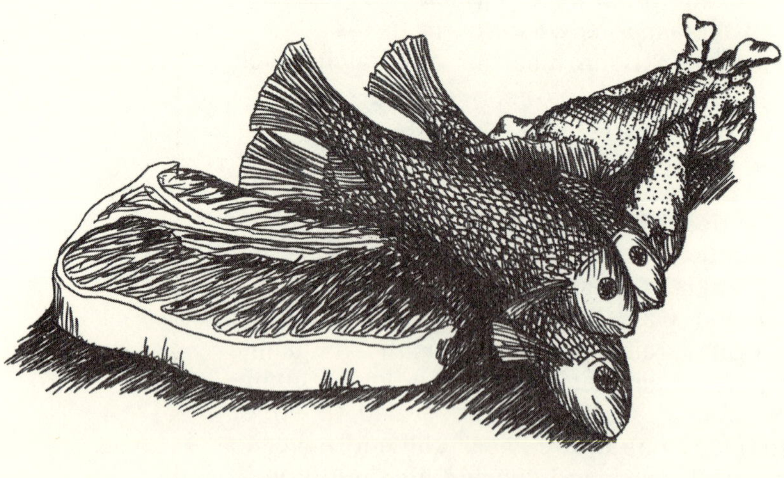

8

Meats, Poultry, and Fish

During America's time of fat and plenty, now closing, meat was counted as a staple protein food, and indeed, it is such a nutrient. A T-bone steak will provide half of the protein an adult person needs for an entire day's work and living. A large hamburger a day, along with other foods, will guard a child against protein deficiency.

However, meat foods have been doing much more for Americans, in the past 200 years, than simply providing us with protein and energy. They are also rich providers of vitamins and food minerals needed by everyone. Steaks, roasts, stew meat, chops, hamburger, liver, ribs, tripe, and sausage are rich in calcium, phosphorus, potassium, iron, zinc, manganese, copper, and vitamins A and B. Needed by all creatures, these food elements are built into the meaty tissues.

So, while eating meats as staple protein foods, we have also been obtaining protective nourishment as a bonus, in the form of vitamins and minerals.

A troublesome fact should therefore be faced: As we cut down on buying and eating meats, due to high prices, we may create new vitamin and mineral short-falls in our daily diets. In the present chapter, we will suggest ways to cope with this meat-food problem.

Low-grade meat often is more nutritious

As dollars shrink and meat gets precious, it is useful to know – first of all – that low-grade meat is usually the most nutritious selection at the meat counter, based on the USDA meat-grading guides. The following table shows this reverse relation between grades of meat and nutritional values:

	Whole Beef		
	USDA Prime Grade	USDA Choice Grade	USDA Good Grade
Protein, grams per lb.	53	58	63
Calcium, milligrams/lb.	31	35	38
Phosphorus milligrams/lb.	485	526	578
Iron milligrams/lb.	7.8	8.5	9.5
Thiamin (B_1) milligrams/lb.	.2	.3	.3
Riboflavin (B_2) milligrams/lb.	.5	.5	.6
Niacin milligrams/lb.	13	14	15
Fat, grams per lb.	161	135	106

Composition of Foods. USDA Agriculture Handbook No. 8. U.S. Govt. Printing Office, 1963.

The food values, except for fat, go up, up, up, as the grade goes down, down, down, for the simple reason that USDA beef grades are based mainly on the amount of fat on the beef critter – while the key meat nutrients are in the lean meat.

This meat fact is shown further by comparing food values in fat and lean pieces of beef:

	Chuck		Sirloin		Hamburger	
	Fat Part	Lean Part	Fat Part	Lean Part	Regular	Lean
Protein, grams/lb.	30	97	20	98	81	94
Calcium, milligrams/lb.	18	54	14	54	45	54
Phosphorus milligrams/lb.	327	971	159	907	708	871
Iron milligrams/lb.	4.5	14.5	3.2	14.5	12.2	14.1
Thiamin (B_1) milligrams/lb.	.1	.4	.1	.4	.3	.4
Riboflavin (B_2) milligrams/lb.	.3	.9	.2	.9	.7	.8
Niacin milligrams/lb.	7.2	23.2	4.8	23.4	19.5	22.5

Composition of Foods. Op. cit.

Again, the fatter the meat, the poorer its nutrient values unless you are a thin person wishing to get fat or an explorer setting out for a 500-mile journey in Arctic climate, needing fat-food for warmth and energy. Admitting that meat fats provide vitamin A and other oil-soluble nutrients, there will be better ways to get these foods in the coming 50 years than buying fat meat at $2.00 a pound in supermarkets.

Meats, poultry, and fish

Lean meats, as a general rule, are better selections at meat counters for most people. Choosing such meats can add 20% or more to the values you receive per grocery dollar. Further to illustrate such an approach, we include an analysis of prices per pound of lean meat from various meat products.

Prices per pound of lean meat from various meat products

Seattle, Washington, market area, September 1973.
Lean meat prices adjusted for moisture content of product.

Item	Price of product	Price of lean meat in it
Beef chuck, bone in	$1.25	$1.64
Beef liver	.97	1.00
Hamburger, regular	1.29	1.47
Top sirloin steak	2.29	3.38
Chicken, fryers	.60	.99
Lamb chops	1.79	2.47
Leg of lamb	1.29	1.72
Shoulder of lamb	1.39	2.18
Pork chops	1.39	2.10
Spareribs	.98	2.30
Bacon, sliced	1.19	6.90
Ham, picnic, with bone	.89	1.33
Halibut steaks	1.30	1.44
Oysters, shucked	1.81	3.70
Salmon, fresh	1.95	2.10
Pork sausage, fresh	1.28	2.78
Pork sausage, links	1.59	3.45
Heat-and-eat sausage	1.63	2.47
Bologna	1.70	2.86
Frankfurters (hot dogs)	1.39	2.28
Italian sausage	1.88	2.45
Polish sausage	1.73	2.25
Liverwurst sausage	1.40	1.78
Minced ham slices	2.38	3.55

Meat grades

Ages ago, when the prodigal son returned to his father's warm hearth after wandering in foreign places, the family rejoiced and killed the fatted calf – not a scrawny, lean one. They knew that fat meat is often tender and has a fine juicy flavor.

It should be remembered, however, that the desert calf for the prodigal son probably would score less than USDA Standard grade today, being fattened mainly on wheat grass and lotus plants, rather than on Iowa corn. Grades of meats are changeable – as are fashions in clothes – and they may be influenced by the amount of grain available to feed the cattle and the costs of grain and meat.

A look at grain and meat prices indicates that it is time to revise the grading system, so more of the meat will be in the price range of present-day food shoppers.

The term USDA Choice is often seen stamped on meats in meat counters and in supermarket advertisements. What does it mean?

This mark means, first of all, that the meat animal was inspected as to fitness for human consumption by the Department of Agriculture Animal and Plant Inspection Service. Further, it means that the meat is of a certain quality grade – in this case, Choice.

Actually, the quality grading is based principally on the amount of fat in, and on, the meat. When a dressed beef animal is at least 34% fat, for example, it may be graded Choice, and marked as such. Many supermarkets pride themselves on offering beef cuts of only USDA Choice grade or better. They do not sell USDA Good beef, which is at least 28% fat.

We believe it is a disservice to customers not to offer the leaner grades of meat. Is not 28% fat meat enough in a land of fat people? The long-term preference for fat meat is psychological and personal, however – we love its flavor.

DES and growth stimulants

Diethylstilbestrol (DES) is a growth and fattening stimulant given to beef cattle, sheep, and other food animals to make them gain more weight on a given amount of feed. Use of DES, it was claimed, reduced production costs in beef by 1½¢ a pound. At the height of its use, in 1970 – 1972, DES was used in the production of over 90% of all beef raised in the United States.

USDA Grades of meat

Most meat sold in the United States is inspected for wholesomeness and graded for quality. Department of Agriculture inspectors and graders perform this service at meat-packing houses and affix their stamps of approval on the meat, with the familiar signs:

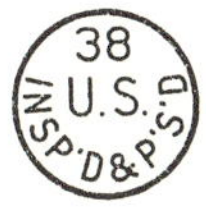

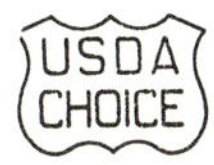

The official standards for meat grades are published by the Department of Agriculture under authority of the Agricultural Marketing Act of 1946. The beef grades are:

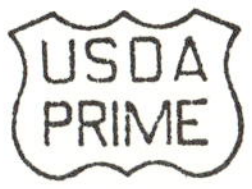

Has abundant "marbling" – flecks of fat within the lean meat – and a generous fat covering. About 39% fat in the dressed meat.

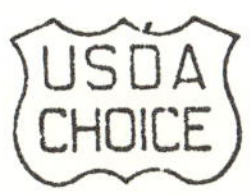

Has slightly less "marbling," but still a substantial amount of fat mingled with the lean. About 34% fat in the dressed meat.

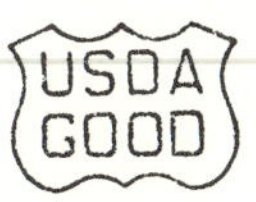

Has still less "marbling" of fat in the meat, but a fair fat cover. Has about 28% fat in the dressed meat.

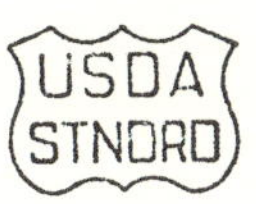

Has little or no "marbling" and a high lean-to-fat meat ratio. About 22% fat in the dressed meat. Always from young animals.

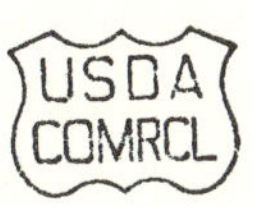

Has good "marbling," but is from mature, older animals. Has about 31% fat in the dressed meat. Good flavor but less tender.

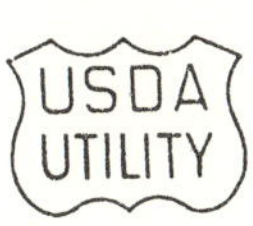

Has very little fat cover when dressed, and little or no "marbling." About 20% fat in the dressed meat. Inferior quality.

The dressed meat is trimmed by the retailers as it is cut for consumer sales. According to the Department of Agriculture, "Each year retailers trim more than 2 billion pounds of fat from the fed beef portion of our cattle production. To the producer, that fat represents an estimated cost of $1.25 billion." (USDA Marketing Bulletin No. 45. July 1968.)

Food flavors

Flavor of foods is a nasal sensation. The odor detectors are located in the nose, and it is here that the chemical differences in the foods are perceived. Olfactory sensors respond to infrared stimuli in the same way the eye responds to colors. Our memory system is then able to recall a mosaic of infrared stimuli and say, "Hey! Scrambled eggs" or, "Gee! Lemon peel."

Since it is unpleasant to take the foods directly into our noses, the flavor factors have to move in the air – as volatile fractions of the foods – from our lips and mouth area to the taste buds. This happens quickly and pleasantly (if the food is good) as we chew and swallow.

Pure starch, sugar, salt, protein, and fats have no volatility; thus, no flavor. Heating, cooking, exposure to air, enzyme action, and bacteria create changes to cause flavor. Small amounts of volatile substances are released, usually from certain oils and fats in the foods.

In addition, some foods contain aromatic compounds of nitrogen and sulfur which we taste and smell. The odor and flavor of onions are examples. Yet, cooking volatilizes onion oils to make new flavors.

Finally, a smoked fish illustrates the effects of enzymatic action, heat, and fermentation during food preparation. A raw fish, if fresh, has

---

Commendable actions by the Food and Drug Administration banned the use of DES in feeds for meat production in January 1973 and further prohibited the use of DES implants in the tissues of meat animals by an FDA order of April 25, 1973. Tests showed that DES causes cancer in laboratory animals under certain conditions and that residues of the chemical were present in many beef animals, creating health hazards for people.

These actions benefit meat consumers even without considering the health factor. The gain in weight and fat of beef animals fed with DES is not a protein improvement or a contribution to the food value of the meat. It is, rather, an increase in moisture and fat – factors that are valueless to consumers.

almost no flavor. When exposed to warmth and air, bacterial invaders produce new compounds, odors, and flavors – mostly unpleasant – announcing putrification. This should be avoided.

To smoke the fish, it is first marinated in salt brine – fully immersed to avoid exposure to air while subtle enzymes improve the tissues. They convert muscle sheaths to gelatin and new protein structures. A mild fermentation, aided by friendly bacteria, occurs.

The process of marination and fermentation may continue for weeks, even months, in experienced fish-eating areas.

When ready, the fish are removed from the brine, freshened, and hung for smoking. This dries the flesh and adds odorifers from the smoke. A waxy surface, called a **pellicle**, is developed during the smoke treatment; this, too, adds odor and flavors. The dish is then ready for a final, cool-smoking (under 90° F), which gently dries but does not cook the meat.

The resultant product, **lox** or smoked fish, is rated excellent in all ethnic diets. It offers primary fish flavors adjusted by fermentation, enzyme action, and the smoke odorifers. Some people add pepper and other spices. In any case, the volatile fractions become flavors, in the complex eating-smelling process called **tasting**.

Also, DES-produced meat often lacks a full meat flavor due to tampering with natural growth processes. DES dilutes the meat and the taste.

Flavor and taste in meats

It is true that flvor and taste in meats are fat-oriented attributes, being derived from volatile oil fractions that are liberated in aging, cooking, and eating the meat. However, there are plenty of fats and oils to generate good flavors in well-produced meats – even when they have only 20% fat. Some of the finest-tasting beef is from old cows, well dressed and cured, although their USDA grade is only Standard, this being a grade with only 22% fat.

Good quality and flavor in meats arise from basic health and fitness in the animal and from good skills in processing and aging the meat. Beef and mutton should be carefully dressed and then aged from 14 to 20 days at a temperature of about 38° F. This fosters tenderizing and flavor enhancement through enzyme action, softening tough tissues and liberating volatile oil fractions that cause eaters to exclaim, "My, this meat tastes good!"

In summary, we suggest a selection of leaner meats in present-day food shopping and discussions with food store managers, encouraging them to stock and sell the leaner grades– Good and Commercial, as well as Standard. This is a good personal food policy, and it also helps the nation get more meat production from its limited, expensive feed-grain supplies. Using valuable feed grains to put blubber on meat animals is fairly stupid in a country of overweight people – one-third of whom are dieting and jogging to lose their excess fat, and many of whom have cholesterol and heart problems.

The leaner meats are more nutritious, and they can be as tasty and flavorful as the superfat grades.

The analogy of milk

Public opinion about milk offers an example useful in under-fifty years ago (1925), milk was sold by dairymen on the basis of its butterfat content and value. When buying milk – in those prehomogenized days – people prized a thick layer of cream on the tops of their milk bottles. Some dairymen guaranteed 5% fat content in the milk, catering to a preference for fat milk among the customers.

Hardly a soul knew that milk is a grand protein food, offering 30 grams of high-grade protein per quart, and that it is also loaded with vitamins and essential minerals. These food facts eventually became known, however, and since 1950, the buying public has been taught to accept low-fat and dry milk products on the basis of their protein and vitamin-mineral values.

Again, a problem is emerging: As milk prices rise to 50¢ a quart for fresh milk, most families have difficulty buying as much as they wish and need. The protein intake per person then must drop, and simultaneously, new short-falls are created in the vitamin and mineral nutrition of many people.

Meats, poultry, and fish

Declines in the use of both meat and milk, due to rising prices, create an urgent need to find practical alternatives in getting enough vitamins and food minerals as well as high quality protein.

Milk is rated among the best of all foods with a protein efficiency ratio (PER) of 2.9. It contains all of the essential amino acid building blocks for constructing good proteins.

Eggs are a similar whole food, with a PER score of 3.5. Eggs and milk are, therefore, able to enhance the nutritive values of less complete foods such as rice, corn, wheat, beans, and peas.

When eaten together with small amounts of milk and eggs, these cereal and legume foods expand their nutritional powers. Synergy happens. A total is created larger than all of the parts.

Poultry – eat an old hen

During 1950 – 1972, poultry broilers (fryers) evolved from dressed chickens in local meat markets into a cheap industrial product. Back then, poultrymen fed young chickens 4 pounds of grain to produce 1 pound of live-weight poultry – a 4-to-1 feed-to-meat ratio. The birds grew more slowly and packed more quality and flavor into their skins. But the price was fairly high. Farmers got about 23¢ a pound for their biras.

The industrialization of poultry production changed this part of the food business and also changed poultry meat. High-speed operators learned to produce 4-pound supermarket fryers (broilers) in 7 weeks with use of only 2 pounds of feed per 1 pound of marketable chickens – a 2-to-1 ratio. This cut the farm price by 40% to 14¢ a pound.

To achieve this result, the poultrymen vaccinate, sterilize, and treat the little birds with various antibiotics and growth stimulators and deprive them of exercise, so the chickens have only one uninterrupted thing to do: grow! It is a highly mechanized process, with birds and feed entering the system, and dressed fryers (broilers) making the exit 7 weeks later as America's bargain-counter meat.

Currently (1973), even with abnormally high poultry feed prices, fryers are 50% lower in price than beef and pork. Dressed chickens in our supermarkets (Washington, D.C. area) are 55¢ a pound; round steak is $1.80; pork roasts are $11.5; and regular-grade hamburger is $1.10 a pound.

America is eating 2½ billion poultry fryers a year – about 10 billion pounds of this kind of meat with a current retail value of about $6 billion.

Is this bargain-counter meat a good buy? Is it good food?

As nearly as we can determine from present-day food research reports, chicken meat, pound for pound, is as nutritious as beef, pork, mutton, turkey, and other meats. The protein value of chicken compared with hamburger, pork, and chuck roast is as follows:

Comparison of protein values and costs poultry with other meats

	Price Per Pound	Grams of Protein Per Pound	Cost per Gram of Protein
Chicken fryers	.55	57.4	1¢
Hamburger	1.10	81.2	1.3¢
Pork butt roast	1.15	65.9	1.7¢
Pork chops	1.45	61.1	2.3¢
Beef chuck roast	1.59	62.2	2.5¢

Washington, D.C., *Retail Prices,* October 1973.

Chicken is a low-cost meat food, compared with other kinds of meats. Beef and pork are a bit higher in vitamin and mineral nutrients, with pork an especially good source of vitamin B. Chicken is, nevertheless, the bargain in meats, due to the assembly line methods used in producing the chicken fryers.

Try an old hen

People who like flavor in their foods frequently complain about the bland, flat taste of present-day chicken – speaking, usually, of supermarket fryers. And they have valid reasons for dissatisfaction. How can a young bird, grown in 7 weeks, develop sophisticated food flavors?

Chickens, let us remember, used to be semiwild creatures, able to walk and fly. They took their time growing bones and muscles and ate a diversified diet of seeds, grains, bugs, grass, and worms. No wonder they had a rich, unforgettable flavor during America's less frantic years.

Francis Moore Lappe says in *Diet for a Small Planet:*

Tips for using meat and poultry to complement the protein in plant food:

1. High amino acid ratings (especially lysine) give even small portions of meat and poultry the ability to complement plant foods, particularly those, such as grains, which are low in lysine.

2. Turkey apparently surpasses all other meat and poultry in it's ability to complement plant protein. Experiments show that if you add only one-fifth as much turkey to a meal of wheat, peanuts, or blackeye peas, the protein quality of the combination will be the same as if the entire meal had been beef.

Some of this earlier quality in chicken can be obtained by selecting "stewing hens" and "roasters" from the meat counters. The cost may be about 20¢ a pound higher, but you obtain a mature bird of good flavor. Also, the hens and roasters can be cut up and fried successfully if you allow sufficient time, at moderate heat, in a covered frying pan. Our procedure is as follows:

Wash and cut up the bird into usual frying pieces.
Chop the breast into about 4 pieces, otherwise too thick for heat penetration.
Mix a beaten egg and 1 cup of milk.
Mix 1½ cups regular flour and ½ cup pancake flour.
Dip and flour the chicken pieces.
Fry at 350°, in covered pan, until one side is brown.
Turn and brown the other side.
Add 1 cup of water (to create steam) and simmer for 45 minutes. Replenish water, moderately, as it boils away.

Turkey meat is an exceptionally fine food to interchange with chicken and other meats. Its protein and other nutrient values are fully as good as in chicken.

In addition, turkey has an exceptional ability to complement cereal foods and vegetables so their nutritional values are increased and enhanced – synergy again. It is explained by the fact that the amino acids in turkey meat dovetail with those in the other foods to make desirable whole proteins – whole foods.

Turkey wings are often an excellent selection of food. They are meaty enough to be substantial. Wrapped in foil and roasted slowly, they become tender and delicious. And remember, added to rice, beans, vegetables, and many other foods, they can tango, since in foods, it usually takes at least two to tango.

Fish – mineral bonus foods

Fish differ from many food creatures in that they grow and live in a water bath. The quality and chemistry of the water, then, influence the flavor and food values of the fish.

Ocean fish, for example, grow in a broth of minerals – the sea water. The water, in turn, receives all of the elements of all life systems of our Earth, from the rivers of land areas. The analysis of sea water shows over 60 mineral elements in dilute form and in biologically interesting ratios. The fish that live in the sea inevitably assimilate the minerals into their tissues and offer them to us when we eat ocean fish.

When eating haddock, salmon, sea perch, sole, cod, hake, clams, oysters, shrimp, lobster, halibut, tuna, and other sea fish, think of this – you are eating 60 food minerals and many of them are useful in your body. The iron will not be high, since seawater does not concentrate iron, but it is the whole cafeteria of minerals you receive when you eat ocean fish.

Fish are excellent protein foods. The quality is superior and the cost per unit of their protein is competitive with hamburger – even at today's high fish prices. For example, the protein in frozen perch is a bit lower-priced, ounce for ounce, than in hamburger.

Adding fish to rice, grains, and vegetables in making whole food meals has been going on for centuries. The arts of doing this are built into the food customs and recipes of Japanese, Polynesian, Filipino, Chinese, Hawaiian, and other efficient peoples.

Fish eggs

Ancient Japanese food customs bless fish roe (eggs) as a superb food. Modern nutritionists agree, since fish eggs have about double the nutrient values of ordinary chicken eggs.

The Japanese are so avid for fish roe that a special open season of only 1 hour a year is provided in some places for harvesting this food. Such is the case for Prince of Wales Island where herring spawn and attach their eggs to eel grass. Entire villages turn out to pull the grass and gather the herring roe. For a large family with many hands making the harvest, a year's subsistence may be obtained during that busy hour.

As the late Dr. McC. Chapman described the price of herring roe, "It is somewhere between the price of gold and platinum."

The Japanese purchase every last salmon roe from the canneries of Alaska. Crews sent from Japan carefully wash, dry, and pack each box so the product will conform to their market specifications. As a result of the Japanese interest in our fish eggs – which we threw away for many years – none are available to the makers of caviar. Hence, red caviar is as scarce as the rare beluga variety from the sturgeon of the Caspian Sea.

Avoid factory-breaded fish, except as a luxury food to break monotonous eating. Federal regulations prohibit breading at more than 35% of the weight of the product. Even so, breaded fish is expensive – usually, double the cost of the unbreaded products.

GUIDES AND SUGGESTIONS

Meat, poultry, and fish

These foods, plus eggs and milk, can serve wonderfully well as "protective" foods, to provide vital protein, vitamin, and mineral nutrients. However, rising prices dictate that they will be eaten less by most people in future years.

As a personal objective, we suggest that you take definite steps to sustain good protein, vitamin, and mineral supplies in your diet, even while reducing the dollar-amount purchases of meats, poultry, fish, milk, and eggs. The following suggestions may assist in attaining that objective.

1. Select leaner kinds and grades of meat. The foods you need are mainly in the lean part, not the fat.

2. Learn about USDA meat grades – Prime, Choice, Good, and so on. Discuss these with your food store manager if he does not offer the leaner meats, and request supplies of such meats for people of your neighborhood.

3. Use poultry as a low-cost meat food, but be aware of the need to improve the feeding practices in producing the poultry fryers.

4. For flavor in poultry, select roasters, stewing hens, and other poultry specialties. They are mature meat and taste better than the 7-week-old fryers.

5. Eat turkey wings. Also, mix turkey and chicken meat with rice, beans, cereals, grains, and vegetables. The mixtures are very nutritious.

6. Choose and eat fish occasionally. It is, generally speaking, a low-cost protein food, rich in mineral nutrients. Mix fish, too, with rice, cereals, grains, and vegetables.

FOODGRAM No. 7

Turkey and brown rice

Do you need new low-cost protein dishes for your family? Then, try a combination of turkey and brown rice. The amino acids (protein-building units) in the turkey dovetail with those of the rice to make a food that is equal to T-bone steaks.

Here is a practical recipe:

2 frozen turkey wings
1 ½ cups brown rice
2 tablespoons cut parsley
2 carrots, diced to ¾-inch size (adjust amount to taste)
1 onion, cut to ¾-inch size (adjust amount to taste)
Water as directed

Thaw the turkey wings and boil them in 2 quarts of water until the meat can be removed from the bones – about 45 minutes. Save the water. Cool and remove meat from bones.
Boil the rice for 30 minutes in the turkey water. Add water, if necessary, so water covers the rice at all times. Salt to taste.
Add the turkey meat, parsley, carrots, and onion. Add water again to cover. Boil for 30 minutes in covered kettle. Season to taste. Regulate water, so the rice and turkey are moist (juicy) when served.

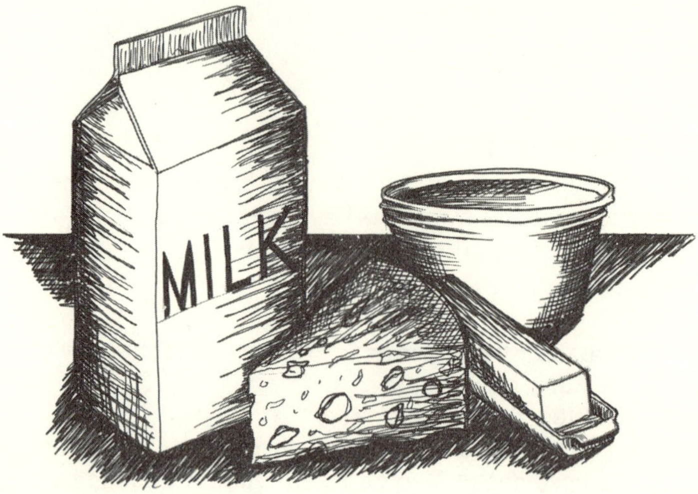

Milk, the life-giver, has been changed since so many Americans moved into large cities. Often, it is produced in distant cow colonies and is over a week old when purchased in food markets. Heavily processed, some people doubt that it is still much of a life-giver. However, milk is a superb provider of protein and calcium. Americans have been getting about 70% of their essential calcium from milk; hence, there is a serious danger of calcium malnutrition as food prices rise and people use less milk. Also, our daily milk has provided complete, *high-value proteins, and malnutrition may occur if we shift thoughtlessly to inferior protein foods.*

We describe the various milk products in this chapter and show which kinds are "best buys" for protein and calcium nutrition. Also, we compare milk with other staple foods and suggest combinations for use in low-cost menus and diets.

9

Milk and Milk Products

Fifty years ago, a Western rancher milked his gentle cow at eventide. While he did this, two cats waited expectantly for new milk. The rancher turned on his milking stool and aimed a white stream of milk at one of the cats – which drank happily, with warm milk all over his face. Then the rancher's boy ran up and opened his mouth, too, for a drink of sweet, new milk.

This might have been called instant milk delivery service 50 years ago when America was half-rural. Back then, even large cities had spacious pasture lands all around them. The dairies were close by, and it was no problem to have fresh-bottled milk on your doorstep every morning, for 16¢ a quart.

Today, the price of milk in Philadelphia, Atlanta, Washington, D.C., Mobile, and New Orleans is determined by the price in Wisconsin and Illinois because huge quantities of milk are shipped from these dairy states into most Eastern and Southern cities. The milk has to be processed and handled in such a way that it can stand shipment for 1,000 miles and delays of a week in reaching market. There are even proposals to pipe milk, like petroleum, from the producing areas into such large cities as New York.

WHOLE FOODS FOR YOU

The price of whole milk is 40¢ a quart (1973), and rising. No price declines are in view. Labor, land cost, feeds, financing, hauling, marketing – all costs are rising. We surely will see 50¢ a quart milk soon. It is permanently a high-cost food, too high for many people to buy and use as in the past.

What can you do to help in solving this personal problem? That is the central topic of this chapter on milk products.

The food values of milk

Milk, first of all, is a protein – vitamin – mineral food, lending itself to a cost-and-value comparison with other protective foods. A pint of milk (2 large glasses) contributes to the daily needs of a moderately active adult person:

90% of the calcium
25% of the protein
30% of the vitamin B *(riboflavin)*

and small fractions of many other nutrients including iron, phosphorus, and vitamins A, D, and C. Often, it is fortified with vitamin D, improving this nutrient value.

The quality of protein in milk, however, is a signal feature. It is complete in the essential amino acids (protein-building blocks); hence, it is a multiplier food – it helps our bodies to capture and use the lower-cost proteins from beans, peas, rice, wheat, and other vegetable sources. A glass of milk with many kinds of low-cost foods will help a child to attain normal growth and learning powers; without the strategic milk, the child will have a nutritional disadvantage when on a low-cost diet.

This is the genius of milk – again, it makes 2 + 2 = 6 instead of the familiar 4.

Raw versus pasteurized milk

Twenty-five years ago, you could open the subject of milk with nearly any group of neighbors and find a strong minority who preferred raw unpasteurized milk and believed it had "unknown" food values not possessed by the pasteurized kind.

Indeed, many people believe this today, and want to buy raw milk again.

Milk and milk products

How about this unknown food value – does it exist, and should it be taken into account when evaluating milk foods?

Unfortunately, from the standpoint of urban grocery shoppers, it is a useless matter whether such an extra value may exist in fresh, raw milk. We cannot keep family cows and milk goats in cities, and state and local laws prohibit sale of unpasteurized milk. Long shipments to market and delays in marketing time, make pasteurization necessary, lest the milk spoil.

Therefore, we will assess milk products in terms of three key values: protein, calcium, and vitamin A. The milk products can then be compared for cost and value with other protective foods such as hamburger, beans, sunflower seeds, and whole wheat bread.

Comparison of milk foods with other foods

Starting with hamburger, here is an interesting comparison of this expensive meat food with dry nonfat milk:

	Price per lb.	Protein Grams per Pound	Calcium Milligrams per Pound	Vitamin A I.U. per Pound
Hamburger	$1.10	81	45	160
Dry Nonfat Milk	.90	162	5,865	130

The dry milk is clearly the better value for the money, with double the protein and over 10 times the calcium for approximately the same price. We show a similar comparison of milk with other common foods in an adjoining table.

If we recognize that milk is mainly a protein – calcium – vitamin A food – and surely this is a sensible view – it is evident that quite a few other foods can supply some of these nutrients at lesser cost. As examples, the following personal or family actions can reduce needs for milk:

- Eat whole grain bread.

- Choose oatmeal and other cooked cereal breakfasts.

Key food values in milk and other foods

Product	Protein grams per pound	Calcium milligrams per pound	Vitamin A I.U. per pound
Whole milk	16	535	650
Skim milk	16	649	690
Dry nonfat milk	162	5,865	130
Canned milk	32	1,143	1,470
Cottage cheese (uncreamed)	77	408	50
Cheddar cheese	113	3,402	5,940
Hamburger (regular)	81	45	160
Dry beans	101	653	0
Sunflower seeds	109	544	230
Whole wheat bread	48	449	trace
Brown rice	34	145	0
Oatmeal	64	240	0
Mustard greens	10	581	22,220

Composition of Foods. Op. cit.

(Eat greens frequently.

(Prepare and eat beans fairly often.

(Eat sunflower (and pumpkin) seeds.

Milk emerges as a high-value calcium food in comparison with many other products. This is noteworthy since getting enough calcium in personal diets has become difficult when one lives in a city and depends on supermarket groceries. A large per cent of Americans have chronic calcium deficiency. This was shown in the Department of Agriculture Food Consumption Survey of 1965 – 1966. It found over 30% of all families with diet deficient in calcium (USDA Household Food Consumption Survey, Report No. 6, U.S. Government Printing Office, 1965 – 1966).

Milk products and how they are made

Dairy milk, as it is taken from cows, contains about 13% solids. It may be pasteurized, bottled, and sold as whole milk or made into many kinds of milk-based foods – the dairy products found in food markets. We will list and describe the principal kinds of these dairy products.

Whole milk is taken from cows and pasteurized at about 162° F for 16 seconds, or up to 185° F for a shorter time. The new ultra-high temperature treatment that may be used on some milk products, sterilizes the milk for 2 or 3 seconds at 300° F. The milk may be fortified with vitamin D by addition of 400 I. U. per quart. If so, this will be shown on the label. Whole milk usually has about 3½% butterfat content.

Low fat and skim milk are pasteurized milk products from which butterfat has been removed. They retain the original protein and calcium values and may be fortified with vitamins A and D and iron. If so, this will be shown on the label.

How cows make milk

Cows are amazing creatures in their ability to make so much milk in a very short time and to sustain the flow day after day. Eating large amounts of food – hay, grain, grass, and silage – they digest it in four stomachs, plus rechewing it once – "chewing their cud."

The rechewed digested food enters the cow's bloodstream and moves to her udder, ready to be precipitated in tiny fractions of milk. Each time the food-laden blood circulates through the udder, small amounts of milk are made and deposited there – waiting for milking time, or for her calf to take it for his dinner.

About 400 pounds of blood must circulate through the cow's udder to make 1 pound of milk. A daily flow of 8 tons of blood is required for a dairy cow to produce 40 pounds of milk a day.

The cow will not give her milk to just anyone – or any calf that asks for some. When she is psychologically ready, a special hormone enables her to "let down" the milk. Her own calf triggers this hormone immediately. The quiet atmosphere in milking parlors, and the soft music at milking time, are signals to the cows: "Please let down your milk."

Skim milk plus milk solids is a milk food to which additional milk solids have been added to raise the protein and calcium values. It may also be fortified with vitamins A and D and iron. This product is sold in liquid form, in bottles and cartons.

Buttermilk, originally, was the milk portion left after churning of butter. It retained the calcium, protein, and solids of cream – as well as small flecks of butter. Present-day buttermilk is usually made by "culturing" skim milk. A culture of bulgur bacteria is added. The product may then be sprayed lightly with milk oils to enhance the flavor.

Nonfat dry milk is skim milk from which all water has been removed. It is sprayed on hot drums, where it dries quickly, and may be scraped off in flakelike particles. "Instant" dry milk is treated with a wetting agent, so it will absorb water quickly when mixed in your kitchen. Nonfat dry milk contains all of the protein and calcium of whole milk. Dried buttermilk is made from real buttermilk – the by-product of buttermaking.

Evaporated milk is made by removing water from whole milk until it is about 50% solids. It is then canned. This process utilizes a temperature of about 240° F. The canned product contains about 8% fat and 26% milk solids.

Condensed milk is a sweetened evaporated milk, based on an old process originated by Borden's in 1856. The addition of sugar and heat treatment make this canned product stable for storage and use in any climate.

Butter is an emulsion of milk fat (80%), water (16%), salt (2%) and milk soilds (2%) – "churned" from cream. You can make it at home by whipping cream until the butter emerges, leaving buttermilk, too, in the whipping dish. The natural yellow color of butter comes from the carotene (vitamin A) in the milk fat.

Cottage cheese is made from pasteurized skim milk to which rennet and a bacterial culture are added. The mixture coagulates, and the curd is separated from the whey by heating. The curd is then cut, salted, and packaged for sale – as cottage cheese.

Creamed cottage cheese is cottage cheese with cream added.

Cheddar cheese is made from pasteurized milk by adding rennet, color, and a bacterial culture. The cheese curd is separated from the whey and "cheddared" into mats 5 or 6 inches wide, then salted, drained, and pressed into large cloth-covered cheeses. These are cured – aged – at 45° F for 3 to 6 months, while enzyme action adds flavor to the product, making typical cheddar cheese. Longhorn, Daisy, and Young American are variations of cheddar cheese. As a cheese family, they contain about 25% protein – about the same as hamburger or cooked pork chops.

Bleu cheese, originally made from goat's milk at Roquefort in France, is made in America from cow's milk. However, a Roquefort bacterial culture (penicillin roqueforti) is utilized, giving our blue cheese the Roquefort flavor. This cheese, muenster, and others are specialty products for people who can afford them.

Process cheese is made by mingling two or more kinds of cheese and adding color, spices, flavors, and other additives. Cream, skim milk, whey solids, and other ingredients may be added in making process cheese food. Federal regulations require that, however, at least 51% of this dairy product is cheese.

Ice cream and milk are simply the frozen forms of milk mixes – flavored, emulsified, and extended into the creamy frozen products. As a usual practice, air is added in the process of "development" of ice cream. The air ingredient may reach 50 % of the total mass of this dairy product.

Butter is an excellent traditional food as a source of vitamin A. Most of the protein and calcium, however, are in the nonfat part of the milk, not in butter. Margarine has exactly the same nutritional rating as milk, and is much cheaper; hence, butter must be classed as a luxury food.

Yogurt is made by culturing milk with bulgur or other friendly bacteria – which mildly ferments the lactose (milk

Cost and values in milk products

Product	Cost per pound	Protein grams per pound	Calcium milligrams per pound	Vitamin A I.U. per pound
Whole milk	$.20(pt.)	16	535	650
Skim milk	.20	16	549	20
Skim, fortified with nonfat solids	.20	19	649	370
Buttermilk, cultured	.20	16	549	20
Cottage cheese	.55	77	408	50
Yogurt	.35	15	503	640
Nonfat dry milk	.85	162	5,865	130
Evaporated milk	.30	32	1,143	1,470
Cheddar cheese	1.30	113	3,402	5,940
Bleu cheese	1.43	98	1,429	5,620
Process cheese		105	3,162	5,530
Process cheese food		90	2,586	4,450
Ice cream	.39	20	662	2,000

sugar) in the milk. It is very similar, nutritionally, to cultured buttermilk. Fruits and flavors may be added.

Value versus cost in dairy products

Value is a deeply personal thing. One might imagine an old Alpine mountaineer, for example, spending his last dollar for a piece of rare Swiss cheese, because he was homesick and this nourished his soul.

Most U.S. housewives do not have that problem – or opportunity. They wish to know which milk products offer good food values for the money. The accompanying table "Costs and Values in Milk Products" can serve as the basis for such an assessment.

We have used the key nutrients – protein, calcium, and vitamin A – for this comparison of values. Other nutrients are present, including vitamins B and C. They may be counted as bonus values.

Several "best buys" are evident:

Milk and milk products

(**Nonfat dry milk** at 85¢ a pound has over 10 times the protein and calcium nutrition of whole milk and skim milk, at only 4 times the price. When reconstituted by adding water, this milk costs only 17¢ a quart, compared with 40¢ for whole and skim milk.

(**Evaporated milk** offers double the nutrition of whole and skim milk at only 50% additional cost. When restored, by adding water, this form costs about 32¢ a quart.

(**Cheese** is still a good selection, offering milk nutrients as cheaply as in bottled milk. Cheddar cheese at $1.35 a pound is, in fact, a better food selection than hamburger at $1.10 a pound. Its protein units are a bit cheaper, and the calcium and vitamin values are much higher than in hamburger.

Back to low-cost foods again

However, the above choices between different kinds of milk and meats do not relieve the basic problem: MONEY. All of the dairy and meat foods have become too high-priced for generous eating every day by most families. New ways must be found to S - T - R - E - T - C - H these high-value foods so they cover more nutritional territory.

The way to do this is to combine them with whole cereals, grains, and breads. The seed foods, too, offer good protein-building blocks, and calcium. Oatmeal and whole wheat (bread), for example, offer good calcium supplies, and milk blesses them with the particular amino acids (protein units) you need for whole nutrition.

Mama can afford to think of this, with satisfaction, when she divides a pint of milk between four children – with their oatmeal for breakfast – and serves whole wheat French toast (slices dipped in milk and a bit of egg). The milk in each case promoted the values of the lower-cost foods.

Americans have been obtaining about 70% of their necessary calcium nutrition from milk and dairy products – and much of the other 30% from cereals and bread. As food prices rise, this is one of the critical points in personal and national nutrition – the calcium supply. Already low, it may be curtailed, with bad effects on health, growth, and vitality. Calcium in personal diets is even more crucial than protein. Most of us are getting enough protein – one way and another – while calcium is marginal. This must be kept in mind in personal nutrition plans and adjustments – in the presence of rising food prices.

GUIDES AND SUGGESTIONS

Milk and milk products

As dairy products rise in price, it may be difficult to buy milk and cheese in usual quantities. The following suggestions may assist in making sound selections among the various products in reshaping your personal food program.

1. Fluid milk. Feel free to select the low-fat and skim milk products. They are fully equal to whole milk in protein and calcium – two of the key nutrients of milk – and the price is sometimes lower.

2. Nonfat dry milk. This dried form is the best buy. When you reconstitute it yourself, by adding water, the fluid milk costs 17¢ a quart – less than half the price of whole market milk.

3. Low-fat milk with milk solids added. This is a new form – skim milk with dry milk added. It provides more nutrition per dollar than other bottled and cartoned milk, and therefore, is a "best buy" at the bottled-milk counter. Hunt for it; often, you will find this product.

4. Cheese. Cheddar, Longhorn, American, and other market cheese products are sound selections. They offer protein and calcium a bit cheaper than bottled milk, and even cheaper than hamburger. Keep the cheeses in your diet.

5. Specialty cheeses and products. The specialty cheeses and cheese food products are not best buys. Their prices are often high in relation to food value. Select them only for variety in your diet. Butter (vs. margarine) is a high-priced luxury food.

6. Buttermilk and yogurt. These are good foods but a bit high-priced for what you get. Count them as specialties to break the monotony.

7. Combine milk products with whole cereals and grains. This is the strategic way to go, if you have a tight food budget. The milk protein offers the jigsaw pieces for making complete foods from whole grains, seeds, and cereals. A bit of milk and cheese, whole grain bread, and good, cooked breakfast cereals can make strong whole food units in your diet.

Milk and cheese in different places

Milk was our food from the beginning. Some people think it is a poor food after childhood. But Abraham served milk to his Divine guests in 5,000 B.C., and Canaan flowed with milk and honey. Hindus used butter long before Christ. Greeks and Romans used it as a salve and hair-dressing. The desert riders of Asia drank horse's milk as an insurance against hunger.

Cheese was invented by an Arabian merchant who carried milk in a pouch made of sheep's stomach as he traveled between two cities. The movements of the camel gently mixed the milk with rennet from the sheep's stomach and made cheese – just as it is done today. Later, each people made its favorite cheeses and some are famous, such as Gorgonzola in the Po Valley of Italy and Roquefort from the caves of France. Our own cheeses from Wisconsin, Oregon, and New York will have places in world history – if the world lasts long enough.

Of all milks, those of reindeer and Chinese buffalo are the most nutritious for land animals. Reindeer milk is 10% protein and 20% fat. If the little reindeer catches up with his mother two or three times a day, he is in good shape.

However, whales have the most interesting milk system of all. The mamma whales have two nipples, just like people, but theirs are set within a layer of muscles and skin. When the calf wants to eat, he pushes his snout against this place, and mamma squirts a gob of thick milk into his mouth. This rich milk may be 40% fat and 12% protein – very nutritious. The little whales nurse for about 6 months.

FOODGRAM No. 8

Good old macaroni and cheese

Do you need a substantial low-cost dinner along about Wednesday?

Then make good old macaroni and cheese. It is no accident that the lusty Italians, many years ago, invented macaroni to fill and feed themselves. It is basically good food, needing only a milkmate to fulfill its struggling proteins.

Here is a good recipe:

2 cups macaroni (whole wheat, golden, or enriched)
1 teaspoon salt
1 cup nonfat dry milk
1 cup diced cheddar cheese
1 tablespoon wheat germ (optional)
pepper or paprika
water as directed

Heat 2 cups of water to boiling. Add macaroni slowly and stir. Add salt. Boil at low heat for 15 minutes, until most of the water is evaporated. Add dry milk, 1 ½ cups of water, and the diced cheese. Mix together. The water and dry milk can be premixed, if desired, or regular whole milk can be used.

Put the foods in a baking dish. Sprinkle top with wheat germ, pepper, and/or paprika. Bake in moderate oven (325° F) for 30 minutes, until golden brown.

This low-cost main dish may be served with a simple vegetable salad and toast or bread.

The nutritional secret is: This dinner has 140 grams of good protein – equal to 2 pounds of sirloin steak – plus 3,000 milligrams of calcium, plus vitamins A and B. After eating it, you feel well fed because you are well fed.

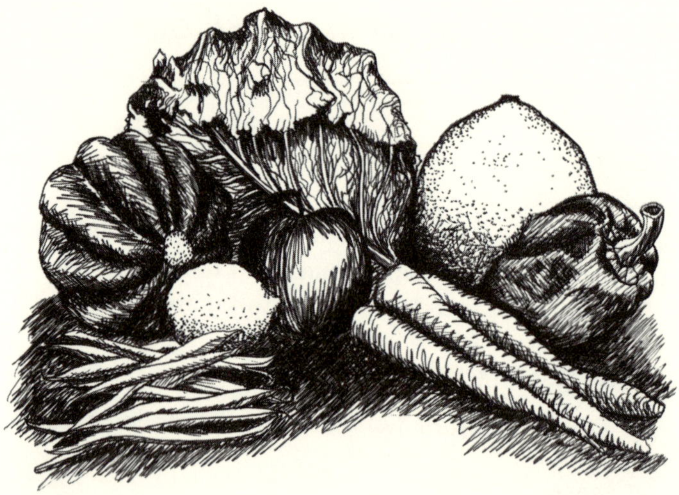

Fresh vegetables and fruits, the traditional foods to protect health, are getting too high-priced for many people to buy and eat regularly. This raises serious questions: "What else will do?" "Are canned goods just as good?" "Are these modern fruits and vegetables up to par in food value, anyway?" We find that lower-cost cereals and whole grains can substitute in part for these expensive foods. Surprisingly, vitamins A and C are cheaper in the form of health food pills than in fruits and vegetables. Getting adequate personal nutrition at reasonable costs may involve the use of cereals, meats, and food supplements as well as carefully chosen vegetables and fruits.

We examine different kinds of vegetables and fruits – as well as other protective foods – in this chapter, and suggest low-cost ways to get your vitamins and food minerals.

10

Vegetables and Fruits

Forty years ago, Popeye the Sailor Man gulped a can of spinach and got immediate power to pulverize his enemies. Since then, millions of children have eaten spinach, and their mothers have blessed Popeye for advertising good food in the badlands of children's foods.

Little did Popeye know that his spinach had 25,000 I.U. of vitamin A and 9 milligrams of iron, and that this was the secret of his power.

In the same era, Sun Maid raisins put their product in little red boxes for 5¢ and asked, "Have you had your iron today?" Ten million boxes later we learned that each box of raisins has 1 milligram of iron and half a milligram of vitamin C. Small amounts, but the raisins tasted good – better than spinach.

We learned a century ago that an apple a day keeps the doctor away; carrots help you to see at night; raw cabbage cures stomach ulcers; pumpkin seeds allay prostate trouble; garlic stops colds; and parsley is good for your spleen.

How about all of this? Are fruits and vegetables essential for health and happiness? If so, what kinds of fruits and vegetables? Must they be fresh and raw, or are canned and frozen kinds just as good? Should they be organic? We will explore these questions in the present chapter.

WHOLE FOODS FOR YOU

With food prices rising, a critical problem has been nagging many grocery shoppers – it may be nagging you: Should we buy any fresh vegetables and fruits at present-day prices, except as luxury foods for holidays and special occasions? Is there enough vital food in these products to justify their cost? Many food shoppers are thinking:

When lettuce is 30¢ a head, I'll buy it – but at 50¢ a head, maybe not.
When juicy red tomatoes are 30¢ a pound, *yes,* but at 50¢ a pound for pale-green hard tomatoes, *no.*
When ripe, sweet cantaloupes are 35¢ each, *yes,* but for hard-meated fruit at 65¢, *no.*

What is in these foods to make them so precious, so dear? Are we buying them for old-time's sake, because America used to be rural and our grandfathers ate apples, peaches, and corn on the cob? Or, are they excellent foods, worth the price even when money is scarce? We will explore these questions, too, in the present chapter.

Vitamin and mineral nutrition in various foods

To get a "handle" on this subject, we will look at the amounts of iron and vitamin A in a number of different foods, to make clear that fruits and vegetables are not the only choices for getting food minerals and vitamins. If they get too high-priced, we can select other foods for vitamin and mineral nutrition – to prevent iron-deficiency anemia and support good health and vitality.

A list of foods is shown on an adjoining page under the heading "Iron and vitamin A in various kinds of foods." By running down the "iron" column, it is easy to see that fruits and vegetables are only medium providers of iron. This would indicate, too, that these products are only medium suppliers of other food minerals, such as zinc, copper, and manganese, since the various elements occur together in foods.

For bargains in iron nutrition, the cereals and grains are outstanding. Look at beans, oatmeal, and sunflower seeds! Meats are good mineral suppliers, too, although expensive.

Iron and vitamin A in various kinds of foods

	Iron milligrams per pound of food	Vitamin A I.U. per pound of food
Vegetables		
Carrots	2.6	40,900
Lettuce, iceberg	2.2	1,420
Lettuce, romaine	4.1	5,520
Lettuce, Boston	6.7	3,260
Collards	4.6	28,680
Mustard greens	9.5	22,220
Garden peas, shelled	8.6	2,900
Green string beans	3.2	2,400
Tomatoes	2.3	4,080
Sweet potatoes	2.6	32,330
Spinach, fresh	14.1	36,740
Spinach, canned	9.5	24,950
Fruits		
Cantaloupes	.9	7,710
Peaches	2.0	5,250
Orange juice, fresh	.9	910
Apples	1.3	380
Plums	2.1	1,280
Raisins	15.9	100
Meats		
Beef cuts	10.7	150
Hamburger, regular	12.2	90
Port cuts	8.6	—
Chicken	5.9	2,260
Liver	29.5	199,130
Fish		
Haddock	3.2	—
Salmon	4.1	—
Cod	1.8	—
Clams	34.0	—
Shrimp	7.3	—
Cereals, Grains, and Nuts		
Whole wheat bread	10.4	Trace
Oatmeal	20.4	—
Dry peas	23.1	540
Dry beans, white	35.4	—
Pumpkin seeds	50.8	320
Sunflower seeds	32.2	280
Walnut meats	14.1	140
Peanuts, shelled	9.5	—
Milk and Eggs		
Whole milk	.2	650
Dry skim milk	2.7	140
Eggs	10.4	5,350
Dried eggs	39.5	19,460
Cheddar cheese	4.5	5,940

In vitamin A, the vegetables offer substantial values, particularly when we choose those with green leaves and yellow coloring. Carrots and sweet potatoes are bargains in vitamin A. Beef liver is sensational, with nearly 200,000 I.U. per pound. When you eat 1 ounce of beef liver, you have an excellent supply of vitamin A for a whole day.

The green-leafed kinds of lettuce are twice as valuable as regular head lettuce as providers of vitamins and minerals. Boston and romaine types of lettuce – the green-leafed kinds – should have a rising demand and use, while the common iceberg type is becoming a luxury – essentially a table decoration rather than an economical food.

Cost of vitamin A in different forms

Pills are cheaper

(This analysis disregards other nutrient values in the foods.)

Product	Retail Price	Price Per pound or unit	Vitamin A I.U.	Cost Per 1,000 I.U. Vitamin A
Fresh spinach	49¢/12 oz.	.65 lb.	36,740	1.8¢
Canned spinach	27¢/15 oz.	.29 lb.	24,950	1.2¢
Collards spinach	29¢/16 oz.	.29 lb.	29,480	1.0¢
Carrots	20¢/16 oz.	.20 lb.	40,920	.5¢
Liver (beef)	$1.09/16 oz.	1.09 lb.	199,130	.5¢
Cod-liver oil liquid	89¢/ 8 oz.	1.78 pt.	400,000	.4¢
Cod-liver oil capsules 5,000 I.U. caps	$1.30/100	1.30 pkg.	500,000	.3¢

Composition of Foods. Op. cit.

However, the main lesson is: Inflation in food prices has scrambled the old home economics guides for selecting and buying fruits and vegetables. The foods you want may cost too much. If so, you will have to look elsewhere in the market for your essential suppliers of vitamins and food minerals – perhaps at the cereal counter, at the bean and pea counter, in the meat department, or even at the health food counter.

Vitamin and mineral pills have become best buys for

some nutrients, in the face of rising vegetable, fruit, and meat prices.

Vegetables and fruits

Currently in Washington, D.C., vitamin A in health food capsules costs one-fourth as much as in spinach and one-half as much as in beef liver.

Such a situation is revolutionary in American foods – almost incredible. It shows that the Department of Agriculture home economists have a great deal of homework to do, advising people what to buy if they cannot afford meats, milk, fruits, and vegetables.

Several vital foods, such as vitamins A and C, have become cheaper in pills than in traditional United States fruits and vegetables.

Are organic foods the answer?

Right or wrong, many food shoppers believe supermarket fruits and vegetables are below par in flavor and contaminated with farm pesticides. The thoughts cross their minds:

Are these products safe to eat, or are they loaded with farm poisons?
Must I throw away the outer leaves of lettuce and cabbage to get rid of these chemicals?
Are these fruits and vegetables nutritious like they used to be?

How can we blame people for such thoughts? Hard, greenish tomatoes, looking and tasting like poor foods, shake our confidence in their nutritive value. Similarly, the stone-hard cantaloupes, avocados, lemons, and plums seem to be inedible. If they are hard and tasteless, can they be nutritious?

No one has answered these questions with reliable research studies. However, about 4 million grocery shoppers have shifted at least part of their trade to health and organic food stores. Last year, they bought over $600 million of health and organic foods – being dissatisfied with super-market groceries.

But, still. Are organic foods the answer?

Organic fruits and vegetables are ones grown with natural manures, composts, and minerals as their fertilizers – without the use of factory-made chemicals and pesticides. They are the old-fashioned kinds our grandparents used to eat, before modern fertilizers and farm chemicals were invented.

The organic groceries are safe; often, they have good flavor and quality. The problem is their high cost – from 30% to 50% more than the agribusiness crops. Even then, the organic farmers have difficulty making ends meet and paying their bills. Labor and hauling expenses in this kind of farming are very high. Big loads of manure and compost have to be gathered, handled, and hauled. The factory-made chemical fertilizers are much cheaper.

We show, on an adjoining page, what has happened to U.S. farming in the past 40 years in fertilizing the crops. The use of chemical fertilizers has risen over 1,800% with no increase in acreage. The food crops are, indeed, being slugged with simple fertilizers that increase yields, but fail to add flavor and nutrition in the foods.

Present-day farming is malnourishing many of the crops, birds, and animals. It is, consequently, malnourishing the people who eat the groceries.

In particular, this kind of high-speed farming is reducing the flow of earth minerals into American foods, thereby curtailing our mineral and vitamin nutrition. It is reducing the real value of the fruits and vegetables in supermarkets – at a time when food prices are rising and we need full nutrition in these foods.

The answer is in restoring balanced nutrition in farming – in feeding the crops, animals, and poultry – not in going back to an expensive 1920-style agriculture.

Many skilled farm advisors know how to do this. Our own earth foods group has many years' experience in growing safe, fully nutritious fruits and vegetables. We know how to do such things as:

- Put twice as much iron in lettuce and string beans, if that is desired.
- Put full color in apple skins, so they are rosy red.
- Put sweet flavor in celery stalks.

§ §

Knocking flavor and quality out of fruits and vegetables

Do organic and natural fruits and vegetables taste better than regular supermarket product? Well, they should. We have done the following things, in the past 40 years, to knock flavor and quality out of American food crops:

- Increased use of oversimple fertilizers by 1,800%.
- Cut down crop acreage by 13%.
- Rubbed out 4 million old-style farmers, and replaced them with large-scale, high-yield farmers.
- Moved 75% of the vegetable production into only four states (California, Arizona, Texas, and Florida), into multiple-crop, mass-farming systems, key-noting high yields at the expense of good nutrition, flavor, and quality.

For fact-minded readers, here are the data describing these trends.

Year	Number of Farms (Millions)	Cropland Harvested (Millions of Acres)	Use of Oversimple (NPK) Fertilizers (Tons)
1934	6.8	344	748,000
1944	5.9	341	1,190,000
1950	5.4	336	2,772,000
1960	3.7	317	5,649,000
1971	2.7	298	13,480,000

The net effect of these changes has been to reduce the flow of earth minerals into the food crops, growing them with an ever-increasing dependence upon incomplete, oversimple manufactured fertilizers.

Economics in production costs have been achieved in this process. However, it is now time to restore a normal flow of minerals into the foods, still retaining efficiency in the farming system.

Food minerals in crops are dropping and the pigs are not doing well

A recent bulletin of the National Hog Farmer reported:

> Spectrometer analyses of over 4,000 grain samples taken in 11 midwest states over just the last four years indicate an unmistakable decline in trace minerals, according to O. G. Rasmussen, an animal nutritionist and director of research for Triple "F" Feeds.
>
> The change in copper alone shows a significant trend, Rasmussen said. "The average copper content in all the corn analyses for the first three years of the study was 2.56 parts per million. But for the last year of the study – 1968 – the average copper content of the corn samples was less than .82 parts per million. That's a drop of approximately 70 percent and it should serve as a warning signal, particularly to pork producers."
>
> What does the decline in trace minerals mean to the individual farmer? Rasmussen cited iron and copper as examples.
>
> "Both these elements are essential in building blood," he said. "In addition to a 70 percent drop in the copper average in corn, we also found that the average iron content of the corn samples for the first three years of the study was 21 parts per million, while in 1968 the average was only 15 ppm.
>
> "To a hog producer, this could mean the development of what is called a stress syndrome, and we have observed this in many situations. Actually it's a blood condition caused by a copper-iron deficiency.
>
> "The hog man may notice that his animals are quite nervous – they may shake and even go into convulsions and die. This condition is magnified if the animal is put under any stress – even that of being moved into another pen.

This decline in food minerals in the Midwest corn crop, during 1965 – 1968, is attributable to higher applications of nitrogen fertilizers, without adequate attention to other crop foods – thereby causing malnutrition of the corn crops.

It causes stress in pigs.

When we fertilize vegetable and fruit crops with unbalanced fertilizers, we may produce de-mineralized human foods, too.

- Improve tomatoes, so they taste delicious and resist spoilage after harvesting.

Vegetables and fruits

Many supermarket managers would like to offer safe, fully nutritious produce, because so many customers are demanding it. They are saying, "If we pay high prices, we want safe, full value fruits and vegetables."

All of this is possible at long-range costs no higher than present costs, since improvements in yields, grades, and keeping quality of the food crops offset the added costs of full-mineral fertilizers and good farming. When the mineral elements are restored in the tissues of fruits and vegetables, the flavor will be as fine again as in the foods of our grandfathers.

This is the sound way to go in American food production, not rejecting organic farming and health foods, but building these good units into a modernized food supply system.

Raw vs. canned and frozen vegetables

The official Department of Agriculture reports show only moderate losses of nutrients in canned and frozen produce, compared with the fresh kinds. Green peas, for example, are about the same – frozen and fresh – in iron and vitamin A, and so is spinach. Canned goods usually have lower vitamin values than fresh and frozen products, but they usually have lower prices too.

Canned spinach has one-third less vitamin A than the fresh kind, but it costs only half as much per pound.

It should be remembered, however, that fresh fruits and vegetables are live tissues, of kinds we have eaten for millions of years; and our bodily systems may be able to get benefits from the fresh foods that we cannot possibly obtain from canned products. Unfortunately, fresh fruits and vegetables are being priced beyond the reach of many people.

Perhaps you have difficulty affording fresh produce. If so, we suggest that you select canned and frozen items, but turn to grains, cereals, and food supplements for lower-cost nutrients. Vitamin A in cod-liver oil and vitamin C as ascorbic acid, for example, can help you in obtaining whole food nutrition at moderate cost.

Food storehouses – in vegetables

Vegetables have quaint ways of storing foods to support next year's seeds. Turnips and parsnips put the nutrients in their fat roots. Carrots do the same. Kohlrabi is more highly inspired, making a round storehouse in its stem.

Cabbages and brussel sprouts store foods in their leaves; cauliflower and broccoli use a sort of flower as their storage site.

Horseradish builds bigger and hotter roots, perhaps with the intention that animals will leave them alone. Radishes make a hot root too, after the tender stage.

Pumpkins and squashes build food houses with seeds inside. When the food house rots, the new plants are fertilized. We harvest the pumpkins and squashes before that can happen.

Some people seem to think the vegetables store these foods for us. However, such thinking is only an ego trip. The plants were here on earth long before we were, and – as things look today – they will be storing foods long after we have departed.

Learn to eat whole fruits and vegetables

Finally, as prices rise, thrifty people can get more food per dollar by eating skins, seeds, roots, and leaves – more of the whole fruits and vegetables. Potatoes and oranges are good examples. Here are the vitamin C scores for these foods:

	Vitamin C Milligrams per Pound
Oranges, raw, peeled	167
Oranges, with peel	319
Increase with peel	90%
Potatoes, peeled and boiled	16
Potatoes, baked in skin	20
Increase with skin	25%

Similarly, apples with their skins have 380 I.U. of vitamin A, while peeled apples have only 160 I.U. Psychology is always a factor and some people despise apple skins. On the other hand, the skin eaters may inherit the earth; and then, everyone will be eating all kinds of skins, rinds, and hulls. It will be the way of life.

Using a heavy-duty blender is a good way to eat fresh whole fruits and vegetables. Oranges can be peeled thinly with a knife, and quartered and blended into a thick, delicious juice of high nutritional value.

When this is done, the cost per pound of orange nutrition goes down, even when the price goes up.

When preparing foods, seek out ways to get a pleasant acceptance of whole fruits, stalks, stems, and leaves. Include some green celery tops in salads along with the stalks, and dice in part of the celery core. Put a few apple seeds in Waldorf salads; it is a sensible and fashionable thing to do. Cook potatoes with their skins on, and teach children the interesting flavor of the skins. Baked sweet potato skins are delicious once you learn to like them.

Remember, liking foods in a learned thing. Otherwise, Eskimos would never eat the eyeballs of caribou, and Polynesians would never eat raw fish. Hot dogs, to many people of the world, are a strange, repulsive food.

Sex and sweet potatoes

Sweet potatoes were accorded the first place among aphrodisiacs (sex stimulants) during the Elizabethan period of English history – and the poets noted this in the literature of the time. For example, Fletcher writes, in The Loyal Subject:

> Will your Lordship please to taste a fine potato? 'Twill advance your wither'd state. Fill your Honour full of noble itches.

And Falstaff says, in Merry Wives of Windsor:

> Let the sky rain potatoes . . . let there come a tempest of provocation.

The shape of the sweet potato may have been the reason people thought it "excited Venus," but, if so, homely carrots would do just as well. A more logical reason for the notoriety of sweet potatoes would seem to be that they were scarce. Imported from Spain, they were expensive, rare, and exotic.

Was it this, or their high vitamin content, that made them sexy?

GUIDES AND SUGGESTIONS

Vegetables and fruits

While farmers learn to grow better, more nutritious crops, and supermarket managers learn to sell them, we offer the following guides and suggestions.

1. Select green-leafed vegetables. The green color in vegetable leaves is formed with food minerals, notably iron and magnesium. You get these values when you choose green-leafed lettuce – romaine, Boston, and bibb varieties – and lower nutritional values from the pale-green kind – the iceberg head lettuce. Choose green vegetables for more food per dollar.

2. Eat more greens. Spinach, kale, collards, and mustard greens are good green foods. When eaten with a small amount of meat, they provide excellent nutrition. Learn to eat greens at least once a week, and you will go far in getting adequate supplies of iron and vitamin A.

3. Select yellow vegetables. The yellow color in vegetables is carotene, the mother of vitamin A. Carrots, sweet potatoes, squash, pumpkin, and rutabagas are excellent foods in this department. If you eat sweet potatoes once a week, you will get enough vitamin A to improve your vision at night. These and carrots should find steady employment in your diet.

4. Eat oranges, plus some skin. The bitter part of an orange is in the outer rind, not in the white part of the skin. So, if you find the taste acceptable, include quite a bit of the skin in your orange juice. Just peel off the outer rind and beat up the rest of the orange in a heavy-duty blender. Add canned orange or pineapple juice if you wish a thinner drink.

5. Also, eat potato, apple, and other skins. The skin foods are almost invariably nutritious; eat them if this is agreeable to your taste. This applies to pears, carrots, summer squash, cucumbers, plums, potatoes, apples, tomatoes, and many other fruits and vegetables. At first, you may do it to get more vitamins and minerals per dollar spent for groceries. Later, you may become accustomed to the taste and prefer the skinny foods.

6. Avoid wilted vegetables and fruits. The fresh produce is alive; it loses vitamin C and other nutrients in wilting. The vitamin A in greens can drop 50% if they are wilted or stored for 3 days at room temperature. Choose fresh, crisp produce if possible.

7. Buy canned and frozen produce on price. The fresh produce is best but often too expensive. If so, choose canned and frozen kinds. When fresh spinach is 65¢ a pound, the canned and frozen products at 29¢ a pound are probably better buys.

8. Avoid livid green frozen vegetables. Some food processors are using a chelating agent (EDTA) to give a bright green color to their products. It is an unnatural green, often seen in frozen string beans. We suggest that you avoid such produce. This chemical immobilizes food minerals and reduces the value of such vegetables.

9. Choose more cereals if prices get too high. If prices of fruits and vegetables get too high, choose more good cereals such as oatmeal, whole wheat (bread), and the seed foods. Also, resort to liver for vitamin A and iron.

10. If necessary, buy food supplements. As we have shown, vitamins A and C may be cheaper in the form of health food pills than in regular supermarket groceries. If so, study the vitamin and food mineral products and prices, and let your good sense be your guide.

FOODGRAM No. 9

Mustard greens with meat

Are you having problems fighting the inflation in vegetable and meat prices?

Then combine mustard greens with meat. Mustard greens are rich and proletarian – a good food for vital people. Pound for pound, they offer more vitamin C than oranges, more calcium than milk, more vitamin A than tomatoes, more vitamin B than corn, and more iron than green lettuce.

When combined with meat, the protein units of mustard greens form partners with meat's amino acids, employing synergy to make a whole food.

Pork is a good meat for this purpose, due to its high vitamin B value, but beef or lamb can be used equally well. Use any good meat that is not too fat.

Here is a practical recipe:

2 lbs. pork shoulder or other meat
½ cup of good quality cooking oil or olive oil
2 lbs. good quality mustard greens
1 medium-sized onion
salt and red pepper

Cut the meat into 1-inch pieces. Wash the greens in a sink of warm water. Repeat washing and draining three times to get rid of all dirt and sand. Tear the leaves to 3-inch size and discard tough main stems.

Heat the oil in a heavy skillet or Dutch oven. Add the meat. Sear it well for 15 minutes, as in making a pot roast. Then put into a heavy kettle (or the Dutch oven) with the greens. Add the onion and salt and red pepper to taste. Soul food people like quite a bit of red pepper.

Stir everything well. Try to coat the leaves with fat to prevent oxidation of vitamin C. Reduce the heat, cover tightly, and simmer for 30 minutes, stirring occasionally. Taste and adjust seasoning and moisture to assure a thorough steam-cooking of the meat and greens. Simmer for another 15 minutes and dinner is ready.

A fair amount of juice will remain in the bottom of the pot after the contents are dished up. This is the rich "pot likker" of the story books. It should be served over the meat and greens, and is traditionally sopped up with cornbread, hopefully made from whole grain corn meal.

This recipe serves six ordinary city people, or four hungry country people.

SOUL FOOD VARIATION

The traditional soul food variation of this recipe is:

3 meaty smoked ham hocks
2 lbs. mustard greens (or collards or kale)
1 medium-sized diced onion
salt and red pepper

Prepare and wash the greens. Put 2 quarts of water in a large kettle. Add the ham hocks and boil them moderately for 45 minutes, using a cover to contain the steam. Add the greens, onion, salt, and pepper to taste. Soul food cooks use moderate salt (1 teaspoon) and quite a bit of red pepper (½ teaspoon).

Cover the kettle and simmer the meat and greens for another 45 minutes, stirring occasionally and adjusting the water and seasoning if needed.

Serve with whole grain corn meal bread.

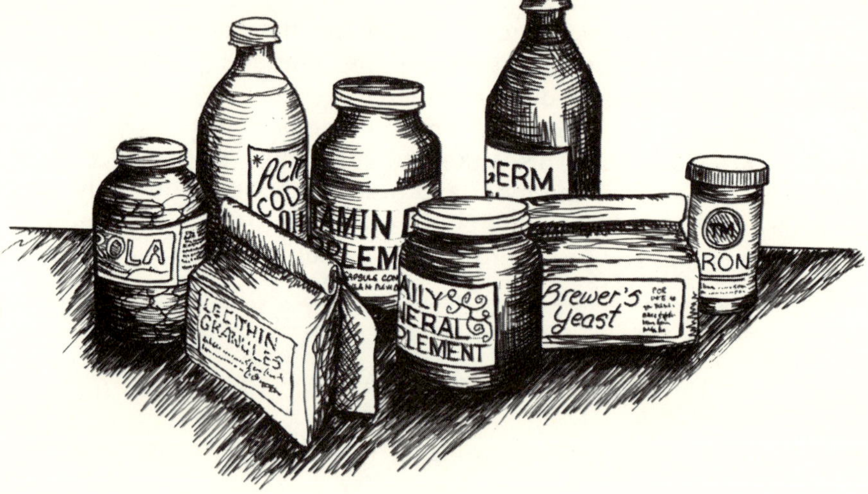

Present-day foods and the styles of eating and living have curtailed most people's intakes of protective nutrients – vitamins, minerals, and raw food oils. Conscious of this, many people are buying and using supplemental foods. *You may be such a person, interested in selecting good food supplements. The different kinds are described. However, the amounts you need will be determined by how well you select your daily basic foods. Eating whole grain bread, raw food oils, and plenty of seeds and nuts* may *provide the critical nutrients you wish and need.*

Eat poorly or only medium well – if you must and when you must – but be aware when you do this. The shortcomings may then be covered with well-selected supplemental foods.

11

Supplemental Foods for Full Nutrition

Sixty years ago, everyone in America ate organic foods, because there were no other kinds. The cows mooed happily in medium-sized pastures. They ate green grass to give white milk for making yellow butter. Then the farmers put straw and manure back on the land to fertilize next year's crops. It was ecological and beautiful. Good cows, good foods, fresh air, no smog.

A carrot was a carrot, was a carrot, was a carrot in those days. No hurry-up farmer in a pickup truck ordered more ammonia-nitrogen for his carrot fields to boost the yield. So the carrots grew on the minerals of the soil and stored them for us – or at least for our grandparents. Same with wheat, corn, apples, lettuce, potatoes, cabbages, eggs, and chickens. Farming gathered earth minerals for the nation's foods – for the groceries in the food stores.

In addition, as we pointed out in Chapter 2, earlier Americans ate much more food everyday than we do now. Consequently, their vitamin and mineral consumption was higher, since nearly all foods contain some of these vital elements.

Good cows, good foods, lots of eating – no wonder the Federal Government decided, around 1940, that extra vitamins and minerals were unnecessary for most people. The food and nutrition advisors said:

> Eat something green, something yellow. . .
> Eat meat, eggs, fish and poultry . . .
> Drink milk every day . . .
> You'll be healthy.

Little did they suspect that such a diet might be too expensive to eat, 35 years later. Or, that high-speed farming and high-pressure food processing would devitalize the groceries.

Or, that 50 million sedentary office workers would be eating canary-bird meals, while 25 million young Americans ate 40 billion McDonald hamburgers, along with a river of sodas and a mountain of potato chips.

All of this – and more – has happened in recent years with the result that America has become a troubled food and health country. One-third of all mature males have heart and circulatory diseases; 30% of all children can expect to have cancer before they die – or die of it; and half of all females show signs of iron-deficiency anemia – a telltale indicator that our national diet is devitalized and undermineralized: short in both vitamins and essential minerals.

It is no wonder that acupuncture doctors are swamped with people whom regular doctors cannot heal, and that the health food business is booming. Mistrusting regular groceries, millions of people have been turning to health, organic, and natural foods, and to vitamin and mineral pills.

What should you select and buy – if you are in this group of health-seeking food customers? We will try to offer sensible guides.

What are food supplements? Food supplements, first of all, are things you eat to fill gaps and short-falls in your regular diet – and they have been on the scene for many centuries. Here are some examples, from years gone by, so we will feel less guilty about our own queer food habits:

Supplemental foods for full nutrition

(In ancient Polynesia, the tribal chief assigned a young lad to gather special crabs and other foods for each pregnant woman, so she would have extra nourishment – for herself and the expected child.

Weston Price. *Nutrition and Physical Degeneration*
Los Angeles: Price Foundation, 1970.

(On the Lofoten Islands of Norway – a place of harsh climate with little sunshine – where people tied down their houses with cables to keep them from blowing away, the eighteenth-century Norwegians placed a pot of cod-liver oil and a dipper by the door. On entering and leaving, they then took a swig of it, sensing that this "liquid sunshine" was essential for their health.

(Captain Cook took 38 barrels of sauerkraut on his great 3-year voyage of exploration in 1773, serving a bit each day to the sailors and all persons on board. This vitamin C food effectively prevented scurvy, although vitamin C was not discovered until 150 years later.

(According to Ernest Thompson Seton, Rolf in the Woods helped young Van Cortland, the Governor's frail son, to win health and vitality. And, in the packet of goods they took into the woods was a rusty nail. Van Cortland put it in a cup of water, and drank a bit every day, to get his essential iron nutrition.

(Our grandmothers doled out sulphur and molasses to their children as a spring tonic. It, too, provided food iron.

(In the same period, herb doctors recommended willow, bark, lily roots, star roots, and mountain grape roots to correct excessive sexual desire.

In our own time, the "chief" is not taking such good care of us – or of pregnant women – so we must gather our own supplemental foods. For some people, this is One-A-Day brand vitamins from the check-out counter at the supermarket. For others, like Bobby Riggs, it is 50 vitamin and mineral pills, 3 times a day. For still others, it is a swig of wheat germ oil, a dish of sprouted seeds, or a dozen raw oysters to "put lead in your pencil."

All of these are supplemental foods – things you eat because you think your regular diet is inadequate fully to nourish you, and keep you well and happy.

We will discuss various kinds of supplemental foods as separate topics. But remember – each food works with all the others, helping them to nourish you. None works alone.

Vitamin A It is an oil-soluble vitamin, received only in oils and fats of our foods. When in vegetable leaves, such as spinach, the vitamin A is in the tiny oil deposits in the leaves. When in fish, birds, and animal tissues, it is in their fat – often accumulated in their livers, as in cod-liver oil.

The following foods that you may not normally eat will boost your vitamin A, acting as food supplements:

Animal and bird livers of all kinds.* One-fourth of a pound of beef liver provides 50,000 I.U. of vitamin A – enough for 10 days for one person, according to present nutritional guides. Pork, lamb, chicken, turkey, and goose livers are all potent sources.

Garden greens, carrots, and sweet potatoes. Try to eat some of each of these vegetables each week. Pound for pound, they offer about one-third as much vitamin A as beef liver.

Desiccated liver pills. These are available at health food stores and counters. If you don't like liver, the pills are tasteless and may serve as a good vitamin A supplement.

Cod-liver oil. Available either in bottles or capsules at health food counters and drug stores. Three or four capsules a day will reassure vitamin A nutrition.

Vitamin A pills, labeled as such. Many health food companies offer vitamin A under their own brand name. The labels show the contents in each pill.

* We are aware that many animal and bird livers are polluted with farm chemicals, and consequently, are unfit to eat. So are many other foods, in some degree. Our whole society is polluted to some extent. But life – and eating – must go on. Try to select healthy, unpolluted foods, including liver. Encourage your food store manager to analyze samples of liver and other foods, so he can *certify* that they are acceptable as human food.

The packaging and sale of vitamin A is governed by Food and Drug Administration regulations, summarized on an adjoining page. As you will notice, if the pill sizes exceed the upper limit of FDA's recommended daily allowance – 5,000 I.U. in the case of vitamin A – the product becomes an over-the-counter drug; and if the pill sizes or suggested daily intakes exceed 10,000 I.U., the product becomes a prescription drug, available only on a doctor's prescription.

Supplemental foods for full nutrition

Hence, the highest capsule strength of vitamin A in many food stores, after January 1, 1974, will be 5,000 I.U., this being FDA's recommended daily allowance.

This is a weird regulation, in view of the fact that a can of spinach has over 20,000 I.U. of vitamin A, freely available without doctors' prescriptions.

Many sensible people rightly believe the doctors and prescription druggists are conducting a public "rip-off," with the assistance of Food and Drug Administration, in this requirement that people get doctors' prescriptions for certain vitamin A products.

Vitamin B

It is a water-soluble vitamin, commonly found – as we have noted in Chapters 5 and 6 – in cereals, seeds, and nuts. Also, in meats, liver, eggs, yeast, and milk. Lean pork is a good vitamin B food, particularly for vitamin B_1; hence, its selection to go along with cooked greens.

Vitamin B is a whole family of nutrients – B_1, B_2, B_6, B_{12}, niacin, folic acid, pantothenic acid, and biotin plus others in the process of being discovered as essential.

The following foods, over and above a conventional American diet, will give vitamin B insurance:

Whole grain bread. If you eat it regularly, your vitamin B needs may be fairly well covered, depending on your individual requirements, and how much bread you eat.

Seeds, whole cereals, nuts, and legumes. Pumpkin, sunflower, and sesame seeds; unpolished rice, oatmeal, granola, familia, peanuts, peanut butter, peas, beans, and soybeans are good natural providers of the B vitamins, reducing your need for other supplements.

Sprouted seeds and grains. These are especially good vitamin B suppliers.

Brewer's yeast. This is an excellent vitamin B food since it offers whole clusters of vitamins and minerals together. It can be added as a powder to blended foods such as "breakfast cocktails," or taken in compressed tablet form.

Vitamin B Complex pills. Available at health food counters and stores; these can cover most other needs.

Recently, vitamin B foods are being used in treating mental-emotional illnesses, alcoholism, and even learning deficiencies in children. Dr. Alan Cott, physician-psychiatrist in New York, is a leader in this field – utilizing specific foods in treatment of mental, emotional, and physical disorders.

Vitamin C

This is a water-soluble vitamin; hence, your body does not store it for future use and eliminates any excess supplies via your body wastes. If you take too much vitamin C, the damage is mainly to your pocketbook, rather than to your body.

The following forms of this vitamin, over and above conventional foods, may satisfy your wishes and needs:

Acerola – the Caribbean cherry. This subtropical fruit collects vitamin C; consequently, many health food counters offer it in various products. It is a good natural source.

Rose hips. These are fruits of rose bushes – the flesh of the rose-seed piece. Interestingly, roses are first cousins to apples. You'll notice that their leaves are similar. Also, both plants put their seeds in a fleshy fruit. Rose hip products can be found in health food stores.

Supplemental foods for full nutrition

Vitamin C Complex with bio-flavonoids. This form of health food pills contains the food "companions" with which vitamin C is associated in nature – notably rutin and hesperidin.

Vitamin C synthetic. This form is ascorbic acid, the cheapest available source of vitamin C.

After the new FDA regulations go into effect, the highest-strength vitamin C pills, except as over-the-counter drugs, will contain only 90 milligrams.

People who wish to follow Dr. Linus Pauling's example of 2 grams a day will then have to take 22 vitamin C (ascorbic acid) pills, or go to drug counters for this food. Again, this seems to be an unwarranted invasion of privacy by the Food and Drug Administration.

Vitamin D

Similar to vitamin A, this is an oil-soluble nutrient found in milk fat, cheese, liver, eggs, and fish oils. The Food and Drug Administration regulates its labeling and sale rather closely.

The oil-rich vitamin A foods, listed above, provide vitamin D as a companion nutrient in a sound relationship for human use. Therefore, good choices of supplements for boosting vitamin D nutrition are: liver, milk, eggs, desiccated liver tablets and cod-liver oil.

Health food stores and counters offer vitamin D capsules, labeled as such.

Vitamin E

This vitamin is oil-soluble, found mainly in seeds and cereals – in the oily parts of these foods. Wheat germ oil, for example, is rich in vitamin E. Preliminary reports indicate that subtle companion factors in vegetable oils may improve the values of vitamin E for human nutrition. Heavy processing with temperatures above 200°F may destroy these companion factors as well as the vitamin E. Hence, raw and lightly processed oil foods are preferred.

Federal regulations governing labeling and sale of dietary foods

The Food and Drug Administration has published new regulations governing the sale of vitamins, minerals and related food supplements. Portions of these regulations are as follows:

A food for "special dietary use" is one:

supplying a vitamin, mineral or other dietary property for use by man to supplement his diet by increasing the total dietary intake, except for foods for which nutrition labeling is used as required pursuant to this chapter.

Any product containing more than the upper limit of the U.S. RDA [Recommended Daily Allowance] per serving [or . . . per daily recommended quantity] of a vitamin or mineral . . . is a drug, except for conventional foods which contain naturally occurring amounts in excess of these limits. . . . (125.1, items [a], [1], [h]. Federal Register, Vol. 38, no. 148, U.S. Government Printing Office, August 2, 1973.)

The term "U.S. recommended daily allowance" (U.S. RDA) means the following daily amounts of the following vitamins and minerals:

Vitamins and Minerals	Unit of Measurement	Adults and Children 4 or More Years of age	Upper Limit for Adults and Children
Vitamin A	I. U.	5,000	5,000
Vitamin D	"	400	400
Vitamin E	"	30	45
Vitamin C	milligrams	60	90
Folic acid	"	0 .4	0.4
Thiamine	"	1 .5	2.25
Riboflavin	"	1 .7	2.6
Niacin	"	20	30
Vitamin B_6	"	2 .0	3.0
Vitamin B_{12}	micrograms	6	9
Biotin	milligrams	0 .30	0.45
Pantothenic acid	"	10	15
Calcium	grams	1 .0	1.5
Phosphorus	"	1 .0	1.5
Iodine	micrograms	150	225
Iron	milligrams	18	27
Magnesium	"	400	600
Copper	"	2 .0	3.0
Zinc	"	15	22.5

(Item 125.1, *Op. cit.* Upper limits column from Item 80.1 [f], [1]. *op. cit.*)

A food . . . for special dietary use shall be deemed to be misbranded . . . if its labeling bears any statement . . . that it represents, suggests or implies: . . . that a balanced diet of ordinary foods cannot supply adequate amounts of nutrients. (Item 125.2 [b], [2], *Op. cit.*)

In view of the toxicity of excessive consumption of vitamin A, the Food and Drug Administration finds that, in order to protect the public health, oral preparations containing vitamin A in excess of 10,000 IU per dosage unit or recommended daily intake are drugs . . . and shall be restricted to prescription sale." (Item 3.94. *Op. cit.*)

A companion order, with the same wording, prohibits sale of vitamin D in dosages or recommended daily intakes in excess of 400 I.U. (Item 3.94. *Op. cit.*)

These orders are in effect, although members of the health food industry have filed legal actions to have them set aside.

The new regulations of sales of vitamins, minerals, and related dietary foods are extensive, and they restrict many sound and good products. However, such regulations are here to stay, and it behooves consumer groups and good food retailers to help in improving them.

* Food stores with pharmacy departments may be able to sell over-the-counter health foods, classed as drugs.

The following may serve as vitamin E supplements:

Raw, hulled seeds and cereals. Those listed above for vitamin B are also good providers of vitamin E.

Seed sprouts are equally good.

Whole grain bread, eaten regularly, will provide good vitamin E nutrition.

Raw wheat germs and wheat germ oil are practical sources. A teaspoon of raw wheat germ oil contains 10 I.U. of vitamin E.

Vitamin E pills, labeled as such, can be obtained at health food counters and in health food stores. Taken with a raw oil (such as wheat germ), the efficiency of these pills may be improved.

Vitamin K and certain other near-vitamins are under study.

When a human body is burned to crips, the minerals we ate are the sole remains – except for metal cuff buttons, glass eyes, and fillings in our teeth.

Calcium and phosphorus will be the larger amounts, since we use these minerals to build our bones. Noticable amounts of potassium, magnesium, sodium, and sulfur will always be there (in our ashes) too because these are nature's intermediate minerals – found in moderate amounts in all living things.

At the bottom of our personal ash heap, and scattered through it, will be found the part of us that helped to build and run everything else, and to make us human – the **trace minerals**. There are at least 40 of these in tiny amounts: iron, zinc, copper, manganese, boron, cobalt, silver, gold, platinum, iodine, vanadium, selenium, and many more.

Iron has won the most attention, since it forms hemoglobin in our blood and acts as the oxygen carrier. When we lack iron, we get iron-deficiency anemia; but other minerals take part, too, in the health of human blood.

Again, good nutrition is indivisible. Dozens of foods take part and a shortage of one – such as iron – often indicates that our food was mineral-poor in the first place. For this reason, enriching bread with iron to prevent iron-deficiency anemia is a doubtful procedure. People with iron starvation are probably starved for zinc, manganese, and a dozen other minerals too.

The answer is to put the whole wheat kernel back into the bread – not just iron – and take a big step toward restoring adequate nutrition in America.

The following foods are suitable supplements to assure adequate trace-mineral nutrition:

Whole grain bread. Eaten regularly, whole grain bread is a superb provider of iron and other minerals, as well as vitamins and protein. Two slices of good bread a day act as a valuable mineral supplement.

Animal and poultry livers. These are nature's richest iron foods. Ounce for ounce, liver contains about 3 times as much iron as whole wheat.

Seeds, cereals, and nuts. These are good providers of iron and other essential minerals. Pumpkin and sunflower seeds are especially rich in these nutrients. Peanuts and peanut butter have good mineral values.

Supplemental foods for full nutrition

Edible seaweed – kelp. Grown in the mineral broth of the ocean, seaweed is a cafeteria of earth minerals. Spectrographic analysis shows that it offers about 60 different kinds including all of them that are biologically active in human nutrition systems. As a food supplement, seaweed (kelp) can act as a broad-spectrum mineral supplier.

Desiccated liver capsules are available for people who prefer their liver in this form.

Iron and mineral pills. The leading health food suppliers offer these products under their own labels.

Health food minerals are available in several forms; for example, iron sulphate, iron gluconate, and chelated iron. Among these, the chelated form is superior, with gluconates next. Simple sulphates and carbonates of the minerals may react with other food elements, becoming useless as foods.

The natural minerals, built into the tissues of plants and animals, are of course the best.

Lecithin

This supplemental food, of rising importance in a land of heart and circulatory cripples, is the emulsifier of fat in human bodies – or anyplace, for that matter. It is the balancer of cholesterol, and there is mounting evidence that people who are supplied with sufficient lecithin in their foods may avoid atherosclerosis and related heart disorders, when excessive cholesterol is the villain causing the disease.

The natural sources of lecithin are raw fats and oils – the vegetable oils. However, as we noted in Chapter 4 on Food Oils, intense processing tends to destroy the nutrient values in the oils – and this applies to both lecithin and vitamin E.

People who wish to restore lecithin in their diets may select the following supplementary foods:

Raw seeds, grains, and nuts. These original sources of raw vegetable oils offer lecithin in its native form. Two ounces a day of hulled pumpkin, sunflower, or sesame seeds, properly chewed and eaten, offer a long step in getting adequate lecithin supplies.

Lightly processed food oils. These kinds are never heated above the boiling point in processing. They are true cold pressed oils. Some health food stores and food markets offer them for sale. Use of these in salad oils and cooking will provide some lecithin.

Lecithin granules and capsules. Most health food stores and counters offer these. The granular form can be added to other foods, such as to milk and fruit juices, to provide a lecithin supplement.

Protein supplements

Present studies indicate that American people consume about 25% more protein than we really need – since we are one of the world's leading countries in eating meat, milk, eggs, poultry, and fish. However, this may change with the steep rise in meat prices. Our danger is in getting nutritionally undemocratic, with wealthy people and credit-card carriers getting plenty of protein while the nonprivileged majority get badly fed.

Proteins are made of 23 different kinds of amino acids, in various combinations and clusters. Chemically, it is like having a chassis to which you can add certain amino acids to form literally thousands of different kinds of protein structures – rather like building Rube Goldberg models with Tinker Toys.

Our bodies can make all of the amino acids except 8 of them – called the **essential** amino acids (because we have to receive them in our foods). Meats, milk, eggs, poultry, fish and cheese are rich in these **essential** nutrients. Wheat, rice, corn, beans, peas, vegetables and other non-animal foods are usually deficient in one or more of these **essential** building blocks for making good proteins. Hence – our danger again – some Americans able to get plenty of animal foods may grow tall and do very well, while the non-credit card majority may get in-

The essential amino acids – protein building blocks

our bodies cannot make these, so we must get them in our foods

Supplemental foods for full nutrition

Amino Acid	Grams Needed Per Day Women	Men
Isoleucine	.45	.70
Leucine	.62	1.10
Lysine	.50	.80
Methionine Cystine	.55	1.10
Phenylalanine Tyrosine	.90	—
Threonine	.31	.50
Tryptophan	.16	.25
Valine	.65	.80

ferior protein foods, dividing our country into nutritional have's and have-nots.

Luckily, small amounts of animal, bird, and fish foods provide those missing Tinker Toy pieces needed to make excellent protein foods. For example:

- 4 ounces of turkey meat added to 2 cups of boiled brown rice makes a whole protein food.

- 4 ounces of fish added to 2 cups wheat or oatmeal will achieve the same result.

- ½ cup of nonfat dry milk with 1 cup of beans will make a food equal to ½ pound of beef steak.

You need not necessarily cook these foods together, but rather be sure to eat them together. Your body will grab the missing amino acids and make excellent protein for growth and human vitality.

This is the whole food route – the key idea of Whole Foods for You – putting staple, low-cost foods together so you can be well fed, even in a Supermarket Age.

We show on the following page a chart from Diet for

SUMMARY OF COMPLEMENTARY PROTEIN RELATIONSHIPS

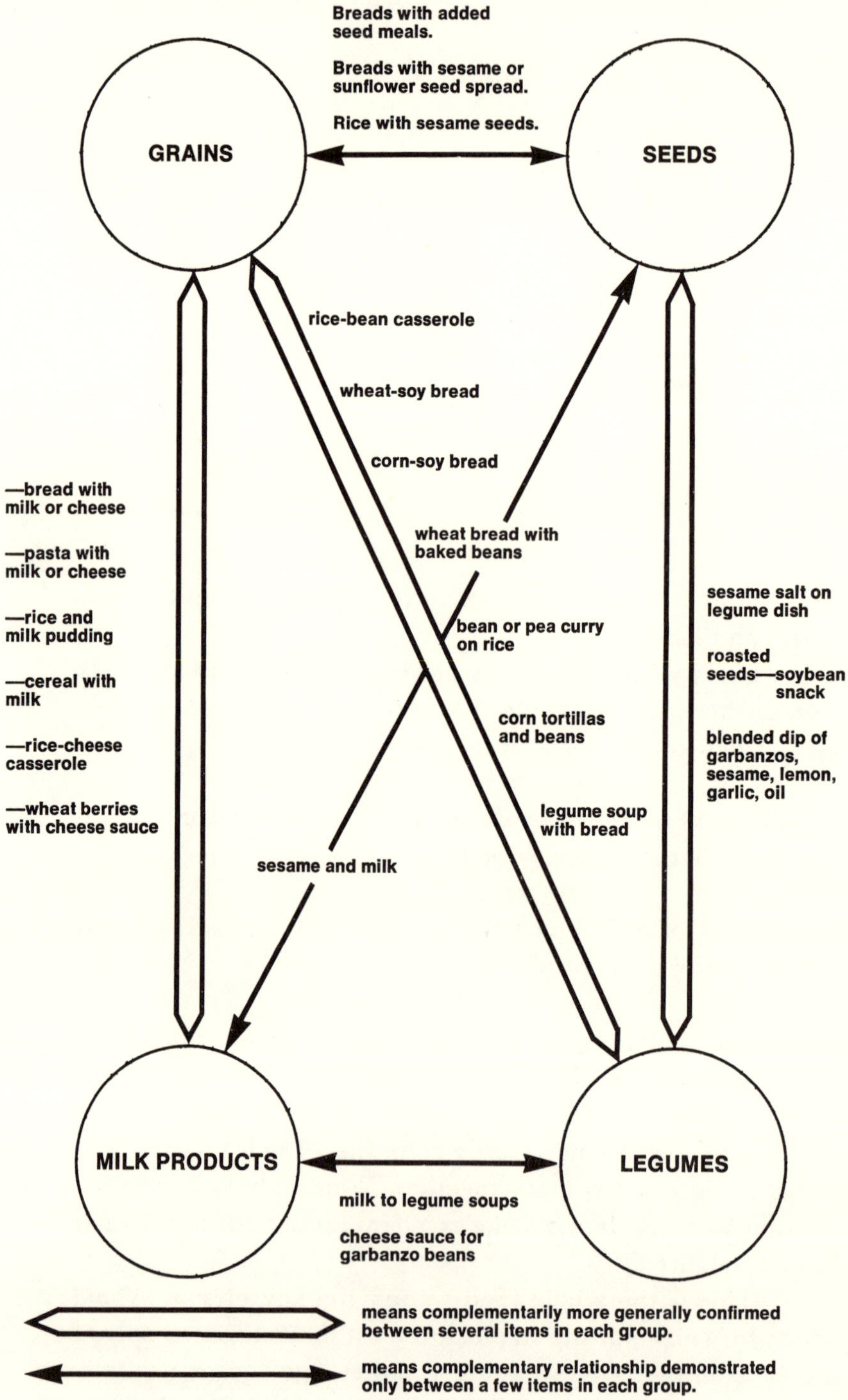

From *Diet For A Small Planet* by Frances Moore Lappe.
Ballantine Books. New York. 1972.

a Small Planet by Frances Moore Lappe, entitled "Summary of Complementary Protein Relationships." Get into a peaceful mood and study it. It shows that grains, seeds, legumes (peas and beans), and milk products can be combined to make complete, high-quality proteins.

Supplemental foods for full nutrition

The same thing can be done using small amounts of meats, poultry, and fish to build good protein foods from rice, wheat, oatmeal, beans, peas, and other low-cost staple groceries.

The finest protein supplements are these bits of animal, poultry, fish, and milk foods, added to regular groceries. For other protein supplements: This chart shows, for example, that skim milk (or whole milk) eaten with rice, wheat, oats, barley, or rye makes complete protein foods. Also, that peas, beans, and lentils are much improved as protein foods when eaten with grains or seeds. Milk products go better with grains (wheat, oats, and so on) than with seeds and legumesbut in some instances, even these are good combinations in preparing protein foods.

Desiccated liver. It offers highest quality protein, and can be obtained in capsule form from health food counters. The vitamin, iron, and other mineral bonuses add to its value.

Protein concentrate. The health food products are made with meat, milk, soybeans, and fish materials.

Suggested supplemental foods

The question is always raised: "How much shall I take?" And, there are always three different answers: "Ask your doctor," "Read the label," and "Try it, and make up your own mind."

Starting with the doctors, most of them have the disadvantage of little or no training in foods and nutrition, plus extensive miseducation from reading Government reports and medical journals. So, unless your doctor is an exceptional person, count his advice along with that of your friends and neighbors. He is a layman in these fields.

The labels on food supplement packages provide vital information. Use it, and build up your own knowledge of these products.

WHOLE FOODS FOR YOU

To help in making up your own mind we include Dr. Roger Williams' guides for supplemental nutrition, from his book Nutrition Against Disease.

These are suggested daily amounts, if you eat a mediocre diet. In our experience, the needs for supplementary vitamins and minerals can be greatly reduced by agreeable selections of seeds, nuts, whole cereals, whole grain bread, and yeast. These whole foods, lightly processed, offer the oil-soluble nutrients – vitamins A, D, and E plus lecithin – the hardest-to-get foods in the entire American diet. They also offer the vitamin B group.

Use these foods generously – offer them to your friends – and eat them with citrus juices and ascorbic acid to take care of your vitamin C needs too.

As a result, you may live to be a very old person, a peculiar objective in our troubled world.

Dr. Roger Williams'* nutritional Supplement guide for the general public

Vitamins		Minerals	
Vitamin A	10,000units	Calcium	300.0 mg.
Vitamin D	500 units	Phosphate	250.0 mg.
Ascorbic Acid	100 mg.	Magnesium	100.0 mg.
Thiamine	2 mg.	Cobalt	0.1 mg.
Riboflavin	2 mg.	Copper	1.0 mg.
Pyridoxine	3 mg.	Iodine	0.1 mg.
Niacinamide	20 mg.	Iron	10.0 mg.
Pantothenate	20 mg.	Manganese	1.0 mg.
Vitamin B_{12}	5 mcg.	Molybdenum	0.2 mg.
Tocopherols (Vitamin E)	5 mg.	Zinc	5.0 mg.
Inositol	100 mg.		
Choline	100 mg.		

* Williams, Roger J. *Nutrition Against Disease.* New York: Pitman Publishing Corporation, 1971. Reprinted by permission.

Producing foods at home is an original American skill – less used recently due to the cheapness of store-bought products. With food prices on the upswing and a scarcity of some staple foods in view, more people will be growing, curing, cooking, and baking foods at home again. It is a good way to get whole food nourishment and to be sure the foods are safe to eat.

We describe home food-grinding and processing equipment in this chapter, and provide suggestions for growing home vegetable gardens, even in cities.

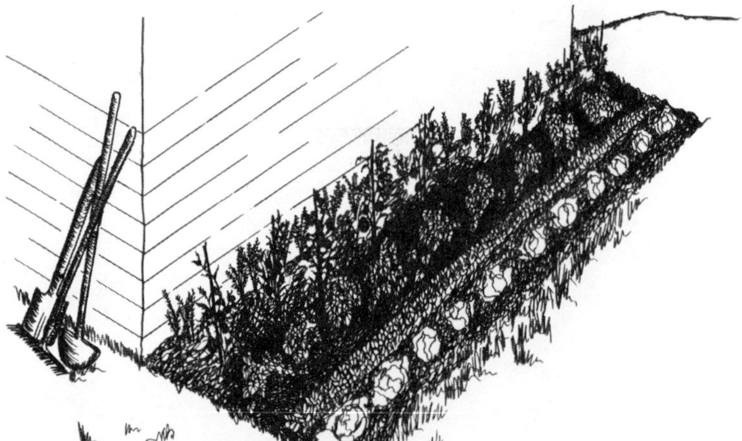

12

Home Food Production

When you produce your own food, it feeds you twice: your ego while you produce it, and your body and soul when you eat it. This kind of food is nutritious, because you make it that way, and it is cheap – much cheaper than supermarket products – because you exploit your own labor and skills.

Take seed sprouts as an example: A homemaker can soon learn to grow $10 worth of foods a week at a cost of less than $1 and 2 hours of labor. If necessary, when food money is short, home-grown sprouts can eliminate the need to buy fruits and vegetables, and they can take care of basic protein and vitamin B needs.

We will explore such possibilities in the present chapter, including growing vegetable gardens, even in cities and on rooftops.

Home food-grinding

In an earlier time, our grandmothers had skills in churning butter, grinding meats, and even making sausage and headcheese. Young lads often helped to grind grain and make apple cider and sauerkraut. The equipment in those days was run by person-power.

Today, good, electric-driven, home food-processing units are available at reasonable costs, within reach of people who seriously wish to improve their food supplies.

The objectives are to get more raw and lightly processed foods into personal diets – more whole foods at low cost. Another aim is to get more fat-soluble nutrients, such as Vitamin E and lecithin, that are so difficult to obtain in super market foods, but are available in home-prepared seeds, grains, and nuts.

The home units can do the following operations quite well.

- Make fresh juice from fruits and vegetables.

- Pulverize fruits and vegetables – pulp, skin, and all – so you can get whole food nutrition from them.

- Grind grains into meal and flour – for example, whole wheat and corn into whole grain meal for making bread.

- Blend different kinds of foods and juices – for example, yeast and lecithin with fruit juices to make nutritious breakfast cocktails.

- Make raw vegetable-oil salad dressing.

- Mix sprouted seeds into food dishes, and chop them up for use in bread recipes.

- Make peanut butter.

All of these operations help the homemaker to get whole food nutrition for the family.

Home-juicing, pulping, and grinding equipment comes in various designs and models – the price varying from $40 up to $500. The chart on an accompanying page describes several examples of home units.

As a rule of thumb, a home food unit should be used at least 3 times a week to justify buying it. Many people use their juice blender several times a day. If the machine helps you to enjoy good foods and better health, it is worth the investment.

Examples of home food processing equipment

NOTE: There are many kinds and brands on the market. These are listed only as examples.

Kind	What It Does	Approx. Price
Acme juicerator centrifugal type	Pulverizes fruits and vegetables and separates juice from pulp with centrifugal force.	$100 to $150
Vita-mix total grinder-juicer. Sturdy with reversible power.	Pulverizes and blends fruits, vegetables, and other foods. Grinds grain. Makes good whole grain flour.	$140
Champion juicer and grinder	Similar to above. Makes peanut butter too.	$100 to $150
Waring blender	Heavy-duty blender to mix and blend foods.	$80
Norwalk juicer and grinder. Hydraulic press.	Pulverizes fruits and vegetables and presses out the juice. Grinds grain. Blends any foods.	$400
Lee Electric Flour Mill	Grinds grains and seeds to make meal and flour.	$125
Hand mills and grinders	Grinds grains and foods with hand-power.	$25

WHOLE FOODS FOR YOU

Equipped with your juicer-blender, you are able to make dozens of whole food combinations. As an example, you can make a breakfast cocktail with the following powerhouse ingredients:

2 cups skim milk
1 egg
2 tablespoons brewer's yeast
1 tablespoons black molasses
1 teaspoon bone meal
2 teaspoons raw wheat germ oil or other lightly processed vegetable oil
1 teaspoon of vitamin C (ascorbic acid) granules
1 tablespoon lecithin granules

Cost—about 30¢. Serves 2 people.

Such a mixture contains enough "jet fuel" to take you off of your launching pad into nearly any kind of a day. Taken with two slices of whole grain buttered bread (toast), it provides one-third of your day's needs in protein, vitamins, and minerals plus cholesterol balancers (lecithin and raw wheat germ oil).

Larger home food projects—scrapple

Making scrapple illustrates many home-food projects that take a bit of effort but yield supernutritious foods. They are worthwhile, even if done occasionally. If you conduct several such projects each month, personal and family nutrition can be improved.

Scrapple is a combination of cereal grain with ground or chopped pork (or other meat), making an ideal high-quality, low-cost protein food plus vitamin B and mineral nutrients. It was invented by thrifty people to use "scraps" of pig meat at butchering time. Today, it can help hard-pressed mammas to feed their families on low-food budgets.

Here are the guides and directions: Buy 3 pounds of pork shoulder; cut out the lean meat. Set it aside. Put the bones and fat parts into a large kettle. Add clean vegetable and fruit scraps – celery trimmings, onion skins, apple peels, anything, except citrus rinds, that seems suitable and nutritious. Add salt, bay leaves, rosemary, peppercorns, and other favorite seasoning. Gently boil the bones, kitchen scraps, and seasoning for 2 hours. Note: You can save food scraps in the refrigerator.

Remove the bones, sieve off the solids and save the rich liquid. Making it was the aim in the first place. Save any meat from the bones.

Choose your cereal. Corn, whole wheat, buckwheat, and oatmeal are all good. Use 3 cups of the whole grain meal. Pour off enough meat stock to use in cooking the cereal to a thick mush. Get this portion of the stock boiling, and stir in the meal until the porridge is smooth. Put it on low heat and stir occasionally with loving care, until thick.

Meantime, back at the range, cut the lean meat into pieces and boil them for 1 hour in the remaining meat stock. Add water if necessary. When the meat is done, remove the pieces, cool them, and grind in a coarse meat-grinder – or cut into small pieces.

Mix the meat with the cereal mush. If the mixture is too thick, add more meat stock. Taste it. Add salt, pepper, chili, oregano, and ten peppercorns – and other seasoning to suit your taste.

Mix thoroughly and pour the thick mush into lightly buttered bread pans. It will be easy to slice when cooled. Wrap in waxed paper or foil, and keep in the refrigerator until ready to eat.

Gently fried scrapple makes the main food for breakfast or any meal.

Making granola and familia

This project takes about the same amount of cash and loving care as making scrapple. The deluxe recipes are given in Chapter 6. They can be modified to suit personal tastes and budgets. If you decide to have a home food-making program, it is advisable to go shopping and purchase a supply of ingredients – good oatmeal, nuts, raisins, seeds, honey, coconut, and wheat germ.

An interesting variation, if you like country experience, is to hunt for fresh nuts in the fall. These may be filberts, hazelnuts, walnuts, acorns, hickory, pecan, beech, or peanuts, depending on where you live. The nuts contain an average of

35% raw vegetable oils – the kind of oil food you need. If you can find a place to gather the fresh nuts, do so and take them home. Dry them with moderate heat over a furnace register or in cloth sacks in any warm place – and use them in your granola.

Shelling nuts is pleasant work, but slow. It is said that a Southwest Indian starved to death beside a pile of piñon nuts because he could not shell and eat them fast enough to keep alive.

Cooking beans and peas

Adjusting yourself in an urbanized society in home food-processing involves psychology as well as economics and money. It can be a protest against the food system, an ego trip, or a practical thing to do. We favor the latter.

In that case, cooking beans or black-eyed peas once a week is a sensible home project. There are many kinds of beans, peas, and lentils and many ways to cook them – boiled, baked, and fried – invariably, they are nutritious.

Pork and beans (or peas) was not invented by the Campbell Soup Company, but by hard-pressed people in places where good foods were scarce and meat was in short supply. They grew a patch of dry beans, butchered a pig, and had a hearty food that tasted good. Only later was it discovered that the amino acids in the pork matched those in the beans to make the whole dinner equal beefsteak. Nevertheless, the miracle happened, and it can be revived by present-day grocery shoppers who are frustrated by high meat prices. Eat beans, peas, or lentils – with a bit of meat or poultry – at least once a week.

Now we are making headway: granola, sprouts, scrapple, peas, and beans. Eating each of these fairly regularly saves enough money for regular meat, fish, and poultry dinners quite often.

Many families will find this to be a sound food policy as meat, fish, milk, and egg prices soar.

beans

Beans, since history was young, have been the poor man's meat – his essential protein to run his mind and help his body to be strong.

They are not good enough – really – lacking in some of the vital protein clusters for perfect foods. But if you have some beans, a few goats, some skinny chickens, and a fish now and then, you can make it.

Millions of the finest peoples of this world have lived this way, producing giants in human compassion, the arts, and a tough ability to live and create – come what may.

The nutritionists say we need about 70 grams of protein each day. Twenty of these should come from high quality sources such as meats, milk, eggs, fish, and certain vegetable sources – notably beans, peas, and lentils. When at least a few of these more complex protein clusters are at hand, our bodies may put combinations together, like jigsaw puzzles, and make fine people of us, if we will only try.

It is the dry seed – the bean or pea – that counts, being almost as good as meat. But beans, like potatoes, are variable.

The beans, as far as we know, were first cultivated by Indians of South America. They were of the kidney bean group, which includes the red kidney beans, the mottled pinto ones, and our white navy beans. The limas, soybeans, and Asiatic mung beans are of other families. Ours are the American beans. Without them, all Mexicans would have died centuries ago – or at least never produced Benito Juarez, Francisco Madero, José Orozco, Diego Riviera, Lázaro Cárdenas, or that fine rascal – Pancho Villa.

These men, and all of the people who loved and followed them, ate beans as a staple food.

Ecological adjustments are quite good with beans. They obey the sun, and follow its light-days in their life schedules. The Montana Great Northerns and the Idaho Reds are wonderful for these areas, but don't yield profitable crops in other places. It is a sunlight thing. The sun tells the bean plant when to grow fast, make blossoms, produce beans, and then die. Further South, the Sun talks Spanish to Mexican beans, saying, *"Vamanos frijolitos cultivanse."*

Beans are like cats. They ignore the farmer's offers of too much care and feeding. They have their own system of using friendly bacteria on their roots to gather foods for them. And – like cats – they will accept some foods greedily, but also thrive on a thin diet.

All of this makes beans one of the greatest foods of all. They will live near you and feed you, no matter where or how you may live.

Granted their goodness, how should we improve and eat them?

We do it differently, by regions. In New England, we sweeten them and add pork, onion, and mustard. Down the East Coast, they increase the onion and add tomatoes. In the Southwest, beans are treated with meat fats and hot peppers, boiled, and "refried," when mashed and heated in oil.

Deep in Dixie, black-eyed peas compete with beans because the easygoing black-eyes will grow almost anywhere. They do well in soils that are thin in lime, where most other legumes would die. And how fine they taste when boiled with fat pork or pig knuckles!

Our way to cook white dry beans or other good quality beans, goes something like this:

> Soak 1 pound of beans overnight. Chop an onion and mix it with the drained beans, then gently boil the beans and onion in fresh water for 2 hours. Use your slotted spoon to transfer the beans to a baking pot, larding the layers of beans with sliced pork or other fairly fat meat. Save the juice from boiling.
>
> Put ¼ cup of brown sugar, 4 teaspoons dry mustard, ¼ cup dark molasses and ½ cup water in a mixing bowl. Stir together and let stand for about 10 minutes so the mustard can develop its personality. Mix with the beans and add enough of the water in which the beans were boiled to cover the contents in the baking pot, lay three more slices of meat on top, and bake in a slow oven – 250° F. – for 3 hours.
>
> Lift the lid, spoon out a few beans and blow them cool. Taste and add salt and pepper to suit yourself. Then finish the cooking, at 350°, with the pot uncovered for half an hour.

Oh, the glorious bean! Its salt-sweet juice is like a fine liqueur, but like its personality, tantalizingly insufficient. You dip and sip and have some more. Enchanting – almost. Satiating – almost. Perfect – almost.

This is the bean – the world's most almost food.

From *Earth Foods*. Lee Fryer & Dick Simmons Chicago: Simmons-Follett, 1972.

Home food production

Growing vegetables even in cities

A debate has raged for 40 years over whether it pays to grow your own vegetable garden – even if you live in the country. When supermarkets came onto the scene, with tomatoes at 1 5¢ a pound, potatoes for 3¢, and lettuce at 15¢ a head, many farmers said, "That is cheaper than I can grow vegetables – we'll buy them."

High vegetable prices and a decline in quality of supermarket produce have changed this. Many city people are growing tomatoes and other vegetables in their flower beds. Stewart Mott, the New York environmentalist, is growing fruits and vegetables on top of the roof in his penthouse.

Nearly anyone can grow some vegetables. Seed sprouts is a good start, growing these in cupboards without any soil. Window boxes and back porches are next – where you can grow lettuce and radishes in soil in containers. Then vegetables in flower beds in backyards – in front yards – and use of empty city lots. And finally, hydroculture (hydroponic) units for serious production of good vegetables in cities – or any place.

If you can manage to get the use of a piece of ground even 20 × 30 feet, you can grow at least $100 worth of vegetables on it – at present-day prices. Four big tomato plants will yield 50 pounds of lovely, tasty, red tomatoes, worth $2 0 by themselves. A flower garden offers enough room for these.

Most of the guides and directions for the garden project can be obtained from library books, seed catalogues, and garden stores. The following suggestions will be useful too.

1. When to spade your soil. If possible, spade the soil in the fall for your spring garden. Fertilize the soil, add peat moss or compost, and spade these in in the fall. The soil will be loose and friendly next spring – better for a successful garden.

2. What to plant. Suit yourself. A good selection for small areas is lettuce, radishes, tomatoes, summer squash, cucumbers, green peas, corn, potatoes, and string beans. The lettuce, radishes, and green peas yield their crops early, and you can use their soil for another planting of potatoes, late corn, and beans – or summer squash. Also, if you grow fall string beans – the climbers on stakes – you can use nearby soil for other vegetables.

3. How to fertilize. Organic fertilizers are, of course, excellent – but high-priced and sometimes hard to get. For the fall treatment, add per 100 square feet of soil: 10 pounds of garden lime, if the rainfall in your area is over 20 inches a year; and sensible amounts of peat moss, compost, or other organic material (dehydrated manure, leaves, and so on). Spade these in with a garden spade or round-pointed shovel.

Then, at spring garden-time, add 5 pounds per 100 square feet of a good garden fertilizer and rework the area – spading this in, plus more organic matter if you can get it. A good garden fertilizer formula is given on an adjoining page. Finally, sow a bit of garden fertilizer under each row of seeds and hill that you plant. Make the furrow, or dig the hill. Sow a bit of fertilizer in the bottom. Cover lightly, and sow the seeds on top, covering them according to directions. This extra fertilizer under the plants will make you into a folk hero – a successful gardener!

4. Seaweed, minerals, and pest control. Seaweed meal and liquified seaweed contain every known earth mineral. When used in gardening, these materials can provide at least basic mineralization of your garden vegetables. And, since your soil has not been heavily farmed, it can offer good mineral nutrition too.

However, the exciting thing about seaweed is that moderate applications help the plants to resist damage by insects and plant diseases. It isn't foolproof – you have to be a good gardener too – but the seaweed is a good measure in pest control as well as mineralization of your vegetable crops. Use ½ pound of seaweed meal per 100 square feet of garden soil, and spray your vegetables 2 or 3 times with liquified seaweed spray, according to directions. You will get superb vegetables, and maybe the bugs will leave them alone.

We have included seaweed meal in the fertilizer formula on an adjoining page.

A full-mineral garden fertilizer

Getting good, full-mineral fertilizers in cities is hard to do, since the fertilizer companies offer mainly the oversimple kinds that are by-products of the petroleum and metal industries. Also, good quality organic fertilizers are getting scarce and very expensive.

As a practical recommendation, we suggest that you go to a garden store or department and select any good organic-based regular garden or shrub fertilizer. A rose fertilizer is usually good, since it will usually contain bone meal and organic materials. It may be of 5 – 10 – 10, 6 – 10 – 4, or similar grade. Get a 40- or 50-pound bag of such a fertilizer for a garden area of 800 to 1,200 square feet.

The fertilizer formula is as follows:

40 lbs. of this garden fertilizer
6 lbs. of dried seaweed meal
2 lbs. fritted trace elements (FTE) or other garden minerals, if available
5 lbs. of Epsom salts (or Sul–po–mag)
20 lbs. dehydrated manure or garden compost
73 lbs. Total

Sweep an area in your driveway or in the street. Pour the ingredients in a pile, on top of each other, and turn with a shovel until thoroughly mixed. Resack into convenient-sized moisture-resistant bags.

Use at the rate of 5 pounds per 100 square feet of garden, broadcast and spade into the soil. Add a bit more under the rows and hills of vegetables. Also, side-dress the vegetable crops with this fertilizer, once or twice, while they are growing – not heavily, just a sprinkle, and water into the soil.

This fertilizer will grow well-mineralized, nutritious vegetables of good flavor.

If you have trouble getting seaweed or garden minerals, feel free to write to us, via our publisher.

Hydroculture – vegetable gardens in cities

The newest thing in city gardening is growing vegetables in protected environments without the use of soil. Such a technique is sometimes called hydroponics, when no soil is used at all and the crops are fed with balanced, diluted chemical solutions.

Recently, this method has been modified, and the plants are grown in homemade soils – for example, in peat moss and sand or vermiculite, to which fertilizers are added.

A good method used at the Arizona Environmental Research Laboratory, near the Tucson Airport, is trough-culture. Simple furrows are made in the soil, and strips of plastic are laid in the furrows, perhaps 40 feet long. The homemade soil mixture is spread on the plastic, 8 or 10 inches thick, and planted to tomatoes, cucumbers, or other vegetables. The plants are then irrigated with a very mild, fully mineralized nutrient solution – keeping the soil damp and growing magnificent vegetable crops.

All of this is done in inexpensive plastic houses, with control of temperature and moisture – truly a modern vegetable production system.

Of special interest to us: Such vegetable units can be obtained in small sizes, and used in backyards (or front yards), or vacant lots or on rooftops. For people who can afford such a thing, it is a good way to get high-quality ripe tomatoes, cucumbers, peppers, lettuce, and other vegetables. The investment cost, however, would be about $1,000 for a 600-square-foot garden unit.

Finally, vegetable plants can be fed through their leaves as well as through the roots. Mineral nutrients sprayed on the foliage enter the plants and may be built into the tissues that become human foods. Home gardening, therefore, offers the opportunity to grow mineral-rich vegetables and fruits – surpassing supermarket produce in this quality. If quite a few gardeners do this and share the good-tasting vegetables with their neighbors, a new force will be created to restore quality and integrity in American farming and food production.

Above all, do not feel inadequate because you have no experience or never lived on a farm. Some of the finest farmers and gardeners are city people who learned very quickly, because their minds were clear – free from rural folklore and old wives' tales.

If you wish to produce more foods at home, use library books as guides, and learn through your own experience.

GUIDES AND SUGGESTIONS

Home food production

The following additional guides and suggestions may be helpful:

1. Grow mushrooms, too. If you learn to grow seed sprouts in your house or apartment, you can learn to grow mushrooms. Just get a book on this subject from the library and follow the instructions. Or, feel free to write to us, via the publisher. Mushrooms are a low-calorie food with a good assortment of protein, mineral, and vitamin nutrients.

2. Use the agricultural services. The U.S. Department of Agriculture is trying to serve city families, since it has lost such a large percentage of its rural clientele, due to elimination of small farmers. Therefore, you can find useful USDA offices in most cities. Look in the phone book under "U.S." or "State Government" for the Agricultural Extension Service Office. They have good home economists and gardening experts to help you in all phases of home food production. Also they offer free pamphlets and books.

If you get frustrated or fascinated – write to us, via the publisher, Mason & Lipscomb Publishers, 384 Fifth Avenue, New York, N.Y. 10 018. We will help you.

FOODGRAM No. 10

Make yourself a soup stockpot

Are you wasting good minerals, vitamins, and proteins by throwing away good food?

Then, make yourself a soup stockpot. It is sort of a cook's compost pile in a well-run kitchen. It catches minerals, vitamins, and proteins from the kitchen scraps and recycles them back into the family foods. For example, the stockpot can capture valuable foods from chewed meat bones, vegetable trimmings, chicken bones, ham hocks, apple peelings, onion tops, pea pods, celery butts, bacon fat, and a dozen other kinds of scraps that were thrown away when hamburger was 60¢ a pound and milk was 25¢ a quart.

It is an honorable thing to do. Good nutrition keeps dignity in people.

Bones are a primary ingredient. They contain marrow, calcium, gristle, sinews, soft discs, collagens, and gelatin, plus scraps of meat; and all of this is superfood to be used in making whole foods from cereals and vegetables. Table bones are good, but you will need fresh ones too, for excellent home cooking. Visit the meat market and make friends with one of the meat cutters. He may understand your needs.

The fruits and vegetables you add to the stockpot provide mild acids to dissolve proteins and lime in the bones, improving the flavor and liberating the various nutrients for you.

To perform the stockpot miracle, get a good-sized kettle – the 2 -gallon size is right for many families. Pack the kettle half full of bones and meat scraps. Add your accumulation of vegetable and fruit items – repeating again – celery butts, onion skins and tops, cabbage leaves, lettuce leaves, snap bean ends, pea pods, potato and apple peelings, cores, seeds, pepper stems, tomato skins, and stray rutabagas, turnips, and summer squashes. Such items can be accumulated in the refrigerator. Omit citrus rinds – too bitter.

Simmer the pot for a long time (6 or 8 hours). This is the temperature just below boiling. Water at the bottom of the kettle vaporizes, rises through the bones and into the vegetables, warming them to 200°. This is sufficient to break cell membranes in the meat and vegetables, so their nutritious contents get out to join the crowd. Avoid hard boiling; use the gentle kind.

Take the pot off to cool at room temperature when this stage of cooking is finished. The cooling will set the fat. Skim it off. Save it for making soups if you need calories and fat in your family. Otherwise, throw it away.

Reheat the soup stock and strain it through a colander. Put the bones and other solids in the garbage or your compost pile. Save the liquid stock. As an alternative, strain the whole mass, including the fat, while it is still hot the first time, and skim off the fat later.

The goodies are in the soup stock, in either case. Let it jell and use it in a dozen ways:

- Eat it straight.
- Cook cereals in it.
- Cook beans, peas, potatoes, and other vegetables in it.
- Use it in cooking rice.
- Make soup with it.

REMEMBER: Happy is the kitchen that has a stockpot. Its people get fed when the others do not.

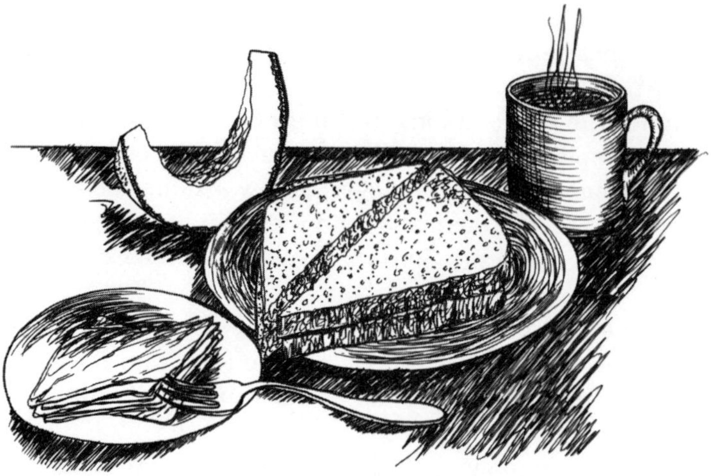

The golden threads of this book run from raw seeds to food oils then to us; from vegetation to meats then to us; and from farms to food crops then to us – via the food markets. If the food oils are poor, we must eat raw seeds, grains, and nuts, lest we semistarve. If the meats get too expensive, we must move down on the food chain and eat grains and vegetables – direct – without using the costly cattle. Living successfully in the coming American years will involve skills in making these kinds of changes – moving around on the food chain when necessary. Meantime, a personal aim is to avoid getting fat, since this is so easy to do in a city-style culture where we are surrounded with high-calorie foods and do little physical work.

We provide in this concluding chapter a summary of the whole food guides, in menus for a week's good eating. Do not be surprised if the meals look lean – we made them that way. Simpler foods – lower food costs – less to eat – lean people – this will be the American Way while we learn new skills in eating, living, and caring for our health.

13

A Week's Good Eating for Healthy People

As we think about good eating, the words have new meanings: First, we should personally like the food – enjoy eating it; second, it should be nutritious – good for our bodies and a supporter of health; third, the food should be assuredly safe to eat; fourth, it should nourish us well – but not fatten us too much. And, as we become city-bound people, with little physical work and regular exercise, it is time to wonder whether people can eat well, enjoy it, and still avoid getting too fat.

As a general guide for adults, we have to achieve good eating on from 2,000 to 2,400 calories a day – and that is a difficult thing for most people to do in an age of TV beer, pizzas, submarine sandwiches, donuts, Danish pastry, french fries, potato chips, blintzes, and happy-hour cocktails. Is it possible to avoid getting fat when surrounded with such delectable calories and cozy places to eat and drink them? Is it better to quit fighting the inevitable – eat, make friends, be lazy, get fat, roll over, and die? Fat but happy – maybe.

Are you too fat?

The eminent nutritionist Dr. Jean Mayer, at Harvard University, is one of America's leading authorities on good nutrition and weight control. He is a practical-minded man. In answer to the question: "Are you too fat?," he says:

Let us first look at the "unscientific" methods for assessing fatness:

> **The mirror test:** Looking at yourself naked in a mirror is often a more reliable guide for estimating obesity than body weight. If you *look* fat, you probably *are* fat.
>
> **The pinch test:** . . . It has been estimated that in persons under 50, at least half of the body fat is found directly under the skin. At many locations on the body – such as the back of the upper arm, the side of the lower chest, the back just below the shoulder blade, the back of the calf, or the abdomen – a fold of skin and . . . fat may be lifted free. . . . In general, the layer beneath the skin should be between one-fourth and one-half inch; the skinfold is a double thickness and should therefore be one-half to one inch. A fold markedly greater than one inch – for example on the back of the arm – indicates excessive body fatness. . . .
>
> **The belt-line test:** In men, the circumference of the chest at the level of the nipples should exceed that of the abdomen at the level of the navel. If the latter is greater, it usually means that the abdominal fat is excessive.

Dr. Jean Meyer. *OVERWEIGHT, Causes, Cost and Control*, 1968, p. 580.
Reprinted by permission of Prentice-Hall, Inc., Englewood Cliffs, N. J.

Dr. Jean Mayer has also said:

> Adapting to these conditions without developing obesity (getting fat) means either that the individual will have to step up his activity or that he will be mildly or acutely hungry all his life.

What do you think of that? Can you imagine 100 million adult Americans getting up from the table "mildly or acutely hungry" for the rest of their lives – or getting to be regular joggers and bicycle riders?

A week's good eating for healthy people

We have a problem. It is understood and felt when we apply calorie measurements to one or two typical American "working class" meals:

	Calories
2 medium—large cocktails	250
1 ounce cocktail nuts or chips	150
Tossed salad with Roquefort or Thousand Islands dressing	190
8 ounce "Branding Iron" chopped sirloin steak (actually, regular-grade hamburger)	530
1 medium-sized baked potato with sour cream and chives—or french fries	450
1 dish mixed peas and carrots, buttered	170
1 small piece of cake	270
1 coffee with cream and sugar	30
Total (oh, my God!)	2,040

Or, an office worker's lunch at Leonardo's Sub Palace, after she says, "I just don't know why I'm so hungry today:"

	Calories
1-foot-long Leonardo's Special Sub-delight, with Polish, Irish, Russian, and German sausage and a bed of lettuce, tomatoes and cheese with mayonaise, chopped pickles, and chili sauce	1,330
1 ounce potato chips	170
2 pickles	—
1 8-oz. coke	200
Total (really?!)	1,700

Such eating episodes, so common now a days, will have to be consigned to the Smithsonian Institution, if lazy Americans expect to survive long enough to watch another 28 years of Monday night football – rather than playing some.

The outline of 21 meals for a week of good eating for healthy people assumes that quite a bit of TV-watching and riding to work is still going to happen – and that only a few of the people will be pushing wheel barrows or laying bricks.

You may have to learn to like some of the foods if you wish to eat them regularly – for example, sunflower seeds for

Can this be you?

For all this, in our society, the woman is physically more active than her husband: she does housework, walks with the children, pushes little carts in supermarkets, windowshops. Her husband, on the other hand, the modern American man, is incredibly inactive. He gets up, and, after briefly standing in front of his mirror using his electric toothbrush and his electric razor, sits down at the breakfast table, goes on to sit in his car, in his office, at a coffee break, at lunch, in his office, in his car, at dinner, and in front of the television set; and, after lying in a warm bath for a while, goes on to lie in bed . . . telephone extensions have been placed in his house to prevent him having to disturb himself. The claims of the American Telephone and Telegraph Company that an extension cord avoids walking 70 miles a year means, by the same token, that the 150-pound person will not expend another 5,000 carlories a year – the equivalent of 15 pounds of fat in ten years.

Overweight, Causes, Cost and Control. Op. cit.

---

breakfast. But do not get put off too early. Try it, you may like it. If you cannot learn to like sunflower seens, try pumpkin seeds, granola, or whole grain toast and a breakfast cocktail. They all achieve the same purpose: restoring your supplies of oil-soluble nutrients – raw vegetable foods of the same kinds your cave uncles ate a million years ago.

You have to chew these foods, and that is a strange new experience too. We know how to bite foods fairly well, such as biting hamburgers and pizzas, but only a few people know how to chew. It is a vanishing skill.

Learning to chew again may help with the weight problem. It takes your mind away from being hungry and requires a couple of calories just getting your jaws working again.

But seriously, changes in personal eating habits, illustrated by these menus, have become a national need. It is doubtful whether American people can reduce their crushing medical, hospital, psychiatric, and dental expenses – or cope with heart disease, cancer, and diabetes – unless they drastically change their food selections and eating habits.

There is no other sensible way to go except in the direction of these model meals. Use positive thoughts; you may learn to like them.

A week's good eating for healthy people

BREAKFASTS

First day: Calories

8 ounces orange or other fruit juice with added vitamin C (see Food-gram No. 3).
1½ ounces (small handful) of sunflower or pumpkin seeds
1 slice whole grain toast and butter
1 cup of coffee with cream and sugar (if you like it that way)

Total 520

Second day:

Same juice, or tomato juice, or other fruit or vegetable juice
2 eggs, however you like them
2 slices whole grain toast and butter
1 cup coffee, as above

Total 420

Third day:

Your selected juice
A dish of granola or familia with milk
Coffee (or whatever beverage you like)

Total 470

Fourth day:

Same breakfast as first day

Total 520

Fifth day: Calories

Your selected juice
1 bowl of oatmeal-cooked cereal with milk and sugar (if you wish sugar – try to break the habit)
2 slices whole grain toast and butter
Coffee or other beverage

Total 490

Sixth day:

Your selected juice
2 pieces of scrapple
1 egg, however you like it
1 slice whole grain toast and butter
Coffee or other hot beverage

Total 460

Seventh day:

A piece of melon
4 ounces of ham
2 slices whole grain toast and butter
Coffee or other hot beverage

Total 530

Total breakfast calories for the 7 days, approximately 3,410

note: On days that you do not eat seeds for breakfast, eat a handful for snacks during the day.

How will you look at age 55?

I am convinced that inactivity is the most important factor explaining the frequency of "creeping overweight" in modern societies. Our bodies' regulation of food intake was just not designed for the highly mechanized sedentary conditions of modern life . . . strenuous exercise on an irregular basis is obviously not advocated for untrained obese persons. However, a reorganization of one's life to include regular exercise adapted to one's physical potentialities is a justified return to the wisdom of the ages.

. . . weight accumulated after completion of muscular and skeletal growth is nothing but useless and dangerous fat.

Even if the same weight is maintained throughout adult life, active tissue is progressively replaced by fat. In other words, even if our body weight does not change, we become progressively fatter as we grow older.

Overweight, Causes, Cost and Control. Op. cit.

LUNCHES

First day: (Calories)

1 medium bowl of soup
1 cheese sandwich on whole grain bread
Coffee or other hot beverage

Total 590

Second day:

1 glass of fruit or vegetable juice
1 serving Waldorf salad or other substantial salad
4 crackers
Coffee, tea, or milk

Total 480

Third day: (Calories)

1 medium bowl of soup
1 sardine or liverwurst sandwich on whole grain bread
Coffee or tea

Total 570

Fourth day:

1 glass fruit or vegetable juice
1 serving tuna fish salad
Beverage

Total 580

Fifth day:

	Calories
1 medium bowl of soup	
1 serving macaroni and cheese	
Beverage	
Total	580

Sixth day:

	Calories
1 glass fruit or vegetable juice	
1 sprouts and avocado sandwich on whole grain bread or sprouts and avocado salad with virgin oil dressing	
Beverage	
Total	560

Seventh day:

	Calories
1 medium bowl of soup	
1 open-faced hamburger sandwich on whole grain bread	
Coffee or tea	
Total	560

Total lunch calories for the 7 days, approximately 3,920

note: Try to limit your afternoon snacks to coffee, tea, juices, nuts, raisins, or seeds.

DINNERS

First day:

	Calories
1 cocktail, if you are accustomed to this, or any social beverage. Country wine is good	
1 serving macaroni and cheese	
Coffee, tea, or milk	
Total	670

Second day:

	Calories
1 glass wine, cocktail, or fruit juice, if you wish	
1 large serving mixed vegetables boiled in soup stock (see Food-gram No. 9 for soup stock)	
2 slices whole grain bread and butter	
Coffee, tea, or milk	
Total	780

Third day:

	Calories
1 glass wine, juice, or cocktail of your choice (or leave it alone)	
1 large serving of boiled turkey wings and brown rice (see Food-gram No. 7)	
Coffee, tea, or milk	
Total	620

Fourth day:

1 social drink of your choice	
1 medium bowl of soup	
1 serving of liver and onions (if you like them)	
1 slice whole grain bread and butter	
Coffee, tea, or milk	
Total	620

Fifth day: Calories

1 social drink
1 green lettuce and vegetable salad with virgin oil dressing
1 large serving of scrapple (or scrambled eggs and whole grain toast if you do not like scrapple)
Coffee, tea, or milk

Total 560

Sixth day:

1 social drink
1 bowl of soup
1 serving, boiled or baked sweet potatoes or baked butternut squash with butter and strip of bacon
1 large serving of mustard greens, kale, or collard greens with meat (see Food-gram No. 8)
Coffee, tea, or milk

Total 640

Seventh day: Calories

1 social drink
1 green salad with sprouts (see Food-gram No. 2)
1 roasted stewing hen* with dressing or steam-fried (see recipe on page)
1 slice whole grain bread and butter
Coffee, tea, or milk

Total 680

Total dinner calories for 7 days, approximately 4,570

* Wrap with foil, so steam will tenderize the hen.

Eating well and staying slim is a whole community challenge

All of these findings eventually bring us to the conclusion that, with respect to physical activity, obesity is in many instances clearly "a disease of civilization." Mechanization and the development of modern means of transportation combine to decrease physical exercise. For many individuals, physical activity is depressed to such an extent that the sedentary state is reached, and excessive calories accordingly accumulate fat.

We eat less, probably, than our grandfathers did. The sight of an old-time wedding menu is enough to demonstrate this point. But, in order to get to the wedding, grandpa had to walk or ride horseback for long distances even in the dead of winter. . . . By the time our grandparents were home, they had expended a large part of the surplus calories they had accumulated.

Overweight, Causes, Cost and Control. Op. Cit.

A week's good eating for healthy people

These 21 meals in a week's eating average 1,700 calories per day – about 119,000 calories for the week. However, they will be supplemented with snacks at morning and afternoon coffee breaks and the piecing that nearly everyone does during days and evenings. For many people, snacking (regrettably) accounts for 50% of their whole day's eating.

Piecing and snacking

We suggest seeds, nuts, fruit, and vegetable juices for snacks. However, we are not Puritans. If you eat well at regular meals, some sins are forgiven in between.

If you get 1,700 calories in your main meals, your snacking allowance – as an average-sized person doing average work – is 500 calories.

Try to live accordingly.

The meals outlined above will provide adequate protein and most of the other nutrients needed by many people. It is marginal in calcium. Try to drink (or eat) a pint of milk a day.

A note from the authors

Nowhere in this book have we advised you: Take vitamin E – it will cure your heart trouble; eat sesame seeds – they'll improve your sex life; or eat whole wheat bread – it will keep you from having gray hair. Nor have we suggested: Take 30 vitamin and mineral pills a day – they will help you to live to be 90.

On the other hand, we applaud the work of many capable health food store managers and clerks who are advising people what to eat and which pills to take in order to cope with their food and health problems. Literally, there is no one else in the country, as a professional group, more capable of advising people in these matters – certainly not the doctors and druggists.

The U.S. medical profession, by default, has turned the food and nutrition field over to quacks, old wives, and curbstone storytellers. Declining to be educated and trained in this field themselves, and being led by elitists who fail to understand food problems, they have become generally biased against selected foods as treatment for illness, and good eating as a way to avoid being sick.

Being so biased, the medical and psychiatric organizations have taken the next step: condemned the use of vitamins, minerals, and other food supplements as a person's means of trying to feel better and stay healthy. U.S. foods and farming, they say, are the best in the world, and if you get sick, it is your own fault.

We do not know a single doctor with a neighborhood practice who is a nutritionist, capable of advising his patients how to select foods and eat to stay well. Nor a dentist with a neighborhood practice capable of helping his patients to avoid dental caries, and softening of gums as they get older.

In fact, we do not know a dentist who uses vitamin C to assist people in overcoming periodontal problems – deterioration of gums and jawbones due to poor nutrition.

Our confessions of ignorance of such qualified doctors and dentists is not due to a lack of medical and dental acquaintances. The senior author has received medical and dental services for over 60 years, and has helped to administer medical and dental services for thousands of low-income families.

Let us be honest and face the fact that most doctors graduate from medical school without ever taking professional training in foods and nutrition. Most of them are no better qualified than cab drivers to advise people about foods – or to use foods and nutrition in treatment of disease.

The country needs legislation requiring medical schools to provide such training as a prerequisite to graduating, and getting degrees of any kind – even podiatrists or urologists. It also needs resolutions by Congress and State legislatures, advising colleges and universities to train school teachers in food selection and the basic facts of human nutrition and advising departments of education to include food and nutrition training in all schools for children of all ages.

There will be five Earth Food books. We hope you enjoyed this first one and will find it useful in everyday ways.

Commencing here – in the food markets – we will soon go back into the American food system to agriculture and the farms, where food crops are grown in the first place. The title of that book will be *Ecological Farming and Gardening.*

§ §

Suggested daily intakes of vitamins and minerals

The Food and Drug Administration has published its U.S. recommended daily allowances (RDA's) for vitamins and minerals used in human nutrition. These are based on the research and publications of the Food Nutrition Board, National Academy of Sciences–National Research Council.

Many eminent nutritionists find the official U.S. RDA's inadequate for certain nutrients, including vitamins C and E, B_6, thiamin, iron, and magnesium. They feel that the research background for these official recommendations is too limited, being devoted to curing classical nutritional disorders such as pellagra, scurvy, rickets, and night blindness, rather than aimed at generating full health and vitality in people – preventing illness in the first place.

While respecting the Food and Drug Administration and supporting its good work in the troubled field of foods, we join with those who find the U.S. RDA's to be inadequate for certain nutrients – notably vitamins C and E.

The official U.S. recommended daily allowances for adults and children, 4 years and older, of vitamins and food minerals are as follows:

Vitamins:

Vitamin A	I.U.	5,000
Vitamin D	I.U.	400 *
Vitamin E	I.U.	30 *
Vitamin C	Milligrams	60
Folic acid	Milligrams	.4
Thiamin	Milligrams	1.5
Riboflavin	Milligrams	1.7
Niacin	Milligrams	20
Vitamin B_6	Milligrams	2.0
Vitamin B_{12}	Micrograms	6
Biotin	I.U.	.3 *
Pantothenic Acid		10 *

Minerals:

Calcium	Grams	1.0
Phosphorus	Grams	1.0 *
Iodine	Micrograms	150
Iron	Milligrams	18
Magnesium	Milligrams	400
Copper	Milligrams	2 *
Zinc	Milligrams	15 *

* Optional in the Food and Drug Administration listing.

Federal Register. Vol. 31, no. 148, Part II.
August 2, 1973.

Earth Foods are those which assuredly are safe and good to eat, because they were grown that way in the first place. And, they have moderate costs and prices, since up-to-date science, technologies, and business systems are utilized in their production and distribution.

Earth Foods I, by Lee Fryer and Dick Simmons, was printed in 1970 to describe such a food-supply system. Interest in the book created the contacts and support for the Earth Foods research, writing, and publishing project, including *Whole Foods for You.*

The research phase is being guided by the new Ecological Agricultural Research Committee, with research units at Clemson University, the University of Maryland, and the University of California. Commencing with processed seaweed, organiform, and full mineral fertilizers, this University-based research is identifying materials (fertilizers, sprays, etc.) that are acceptable in "ecological farming," gardening, and food production. Dr. T. L. Senn, head of the Horticulture Department, Clemson University, is Chairman of the Ecological Agricultural Research Committee. Lee Fryer serves as its Secretary.

Five Earth Foods books are currently being written and published:

Whole Foods for You
Supplemental Foods
Ecological Farming and Gardening
The Seaweed Story
Earth Foods (rewritten and updated)

Whole Foods for You, as the first in this cluster of books, will be read by millions of Americans who have *food problems.* It will help in creating a better food system in which assuredly safe, nutritious foods can be obtained by everyone at moderate costs.

EARTH
FOODS